Mental Retardation and Sterilization

A PROBLEM OF COMPETENCY AND PATERNALISM

THE HASTINGS CENTER SERIES IN ETHICS

ETHICS TEACHING IN HIGHER EDUCATION
Edited by Daniel Callahan and Sissela Bok

MENTAL RETARDATION AND STERILIZATION
A Problem of Competency and Paternalism
Edited by Ruth Macklin and Willard Gaylin

THE ROOTS OF ETHICS: Science, Religion, and Values
Edited by Daniel Callahan and H. Tristram Engelhardt, Jr.

ETHICS IN HARD TIMES
Edited by Arthur L. Caplan and Daniel Callahan

VIOLENCE AND THE POLITICS OF RESEARCH
Edited by Willard Gaylin, Ruth Macklin, and Tabitha M. Powledge

Mental Retardation and Sterilization

A PROBLEM OF COMPETENCY AND PATERNALISM

Edited by

Ruth Macklin

Albert Einstein College of Medicine
Bronx, New York

and

Willard Gaylin

The Hastings Center
Hastings-on-Hudson, New York

PLENUM PRESS • NEW YORK AND LONDON

Library of Congress Cataloging in Publication Data

Main entry under title:

Mental retardation and sterilization.

(Hastings Center series in ethics)
Includes bibliographical references and index.
1. Mentally handicapped—Civil rights—United States. 2. Sterilization, Eugenic—United States. 3. Sterilization, Eugenic—Law and legislation—United States. 4. Medical ethics—United States. I. Macklin, Ruth, 1938- . II. Gaylin, Willard. III. Series. [DNLM: 1. Sterilization, Sexual. 2. Sterilization, Involuntary. 3. Mental retardation. HV 4989 M549]
HV3006.A4M43 323.3 81-7393
ISBN 978-1-4684-3925-0 ISBN 978-1-4684-3923-6 (eBook)
DOI 10.1007/978-1-4684-3923-6

Softcover reprint of the hardcover 1st edition 1981

Institute of Society, Ethics, and the Life Sciences
360 Broadway, Hastings-on-Hudson, New York 10706

Plenum Press, New York
A Division of Plenum Publishing Corporation
233 Spring Street, New York, N.Y. 10013

Participants 1976–1978

GLENN AFFLECK, Ph. D., Assistant Professor of Psychiatry and Pediatrics, University of Connecticut School of Medicine, Farmington, Connecticut 06032

MICHAEL D. BAYLES, Ph.D., Director, Westminster Institute for Ethics and Human Values, Professor of Philosophy, University of Western Ontario, London, Canada N6G 2M2

BURTON BLATT, Ph.D., Centennial Professor and Dean, Syracuse University School of Education, 150 Marshall Street, Syracuse, New York 13210

ROBERT A. BURT, LL.B., Professor of Law, Yale University School of Law, New Haven, Connecticut 06520

JAMES D. CLEMENTS, M.D., Assistant Medical Director for Mental Retardation, Division of Mental Health and Mental Retardation, Georgia Department of Human Resources, Atlanta, Georgia

GUNNAR DYBWAD, Ph.D., Professor Emeritus of Human Development, Florence Heller Graduate School, Brandeis University, Waltham, Massachusetts 02154

HAROLD EDGAR, LL.B., Professor of Law, Columbia University School of Law, 435 West 116th Street, New York, New York 10027

PAUL FRIEDMAN, LL.B., Managing Attorney, Mental Health Law Project, 1220 Nineteenth Street, NW, Washington DC 20036

HERBERT GOLDSTEIN, Ed.D., Director, Curriculum Research and Development Center in Mental Retardation, New York University, Shimkin Hall, Rm. 1032, 50 West 4th Street, New York, New York 10003

JANE R. MERCER, Ph.D., Professor of Sociology, University of California, Riverside, Riverside, California 92502

ROBERT MICHELS, M.D., Barklie McKee Henry Professor and Chairman, Department of Psychiatry, Cornell University Medical College, Psychiatrist-in-Chief, The New York Hospital, 525 East 68th Street, New York, New York 10021

ROBERT NEVILLE, Ph.D., Professor of Philosophy and Religious Studies, State University of New York at Stony Brook, Stony Brook, New York 11794

PHILIP ROOS, Ph.D., National Executive Director, Association for Retarded Citizens, 2709 Avenue E East, Arlington, Texas 76011

JAMES M. SMITH, Ph.D., Professor of Philosophy, California State University, Fresno, Fresno, California 93710

TRAVIS THOMPSON, Ph.D., Professor, Departments of Psychiatry and Psychology, Adjunct Professor, Department of Special Education, University of Minnesota, Minneapolis, Minnesota 55455

DANIEL I. WIKLER, Ph.D., Assistant Professor and Kennedy Scholar, Program in Medical Ethics, School of Medicine, Department of Philosophy, University of Wisconsin, Madison, Wisconsin 53711

Preface

This book is the product of a one-year project[1] conducted by the Hastings Center, Institute of Society, Ethics and the Life Sciences, during 1976–1977. The Behavior Control Research Group—an ongoing, interdisciplinary working group composed of philosophers, psychiatrists, psychologists, social scientists, and lawyers—met four times over the course of the year with special consultants with expertise in the field of mental retardation. At those meetings, participants gave informal presentations, which were followed by group discussion. As the project progressed, formal papers were delivered and subjected to further critical commentary. This volume, in two related parts, represents the deliberations of the group as a whole, and then offers individual papers prepared by some scholars in order to give a sense of the kind of specific arguments on which the general conclusions were based.

We undertook the project to examine: (1) questions of competence and consent; and (2) the practical implications,

[1]The project, entitled "Ethical Issues in the Care and Treatment of the Mildly Mentally Retarded," was supported by the EVIST program of the National Science Foundation under Grant No. 0SS76-14793. Any Opinions, findings, conclusions, or recommendations expressed herein are those of the authors and do not necessarily reflect the views of the National Science Foundation.

in terms of care and treatment, that evolve from differing definitions and models applied to mental retardation. Our study incorporated a range of empirical data on the undisputed facts of mental retardation, a continuous dialogue about factual and theoretical matters on which the experts disagree, a look at the major court decisions and statutes pertinent to our proposed case study on sterilization of the retarded, and a normative inquiry into such topics as labeling and educating the retarded, testing their competence, and ensuring their basic human rights.

We began by posing the following questions: On what basis are retarded people deemed incompetent or possessed of only limited competence? Surely, not all retarded persons have equal capabilities. How ought we assess the competencies of the retarded as they bear on the right to vote, to enter into legal contracts, to rear children? What stance should society take toward the retarded: one of paternalistic intervention? enhancement of autonomy?

The answers to these and related questions are clearer when we consider the severely retarded rather than the mildly mentally retarded. Nonetheless—or perhaps for that very reason—we decided to focus our attention on the mildly mentally retarded, for whom the boundary between competence and incompetence, autonomy and dependence, is much more difficult to elucidate. So, even before undertaking the year's work, we recognized that because our population was the mildly mentally retarded the decisions that must be made regarding special educational and treatment programs would involve issues of such complexity that caution and conservatism were essential. We chose the issue of sterilization as a case study for this project primarily out of the need to supply a narrow focus for the general problems of the treatment of the retarded—and in part because of the recent reversal of earlier social and legal trends.

Sterilization of the retarded—whether voluntary or involuntary—brings to the fore such problems as: how to determine their competence to grant consent for such a procedure; whether sterilization might serve to enhance rather than to diminish their autonomy; as well as the broader issue of their competence to raise children. The first half of the year was devoted to a clarification of the general issues. In the second half we applied what we had learned to two specific issues: the competence of the mildly retarded to raise children, on the one hand; and to grant their competent consent for sterilization, on the other.

The yearlong project was divided into four topics. The first topic explored was competence and coercion. The issue of competence was analyzed through its relevant philosophical, psychological, and legal dimensions. These discussions are summarized in Chapters 1 and 4, as well as in a formal paper that appears as Chapter 10 in Part II. The summary cannot possibly do justice to the anguish, outrage, and frustration we experienced as we attempted to realize a consensus. In addition, disagreement arose among group members as to whether and according to what criteria the mildly mentally retarded can be distinguished from the normal population. Several different positions were advanced, and the elements of that debate are captured in Chapters 1 and 2.

Our second concern was: Who are the retarded and what are their capabilities? The group addressed the following questions: How do the retarded differ from normal people? What are the implications of these differences for the capability to perform various tasks and for attributing dependent status to the mildly mentally retarded? What are the purposes and justifications of intervention with the mildly mentally retarded? Various theoretical models of the definition and nature of mental retardation were discussed—legal, psychological, sociological—and it became apparent that the definition of retardation would itself bias the arguments concerning its treatment. Presentations ranged in perspective from the cognitive-developmental, emphasizing the differences in the achievement of various stages of development between retarded and normal children, to—in sharp disagreement—the sociological, maintaining that the labeling of certain children as mentally retarded is an artifact of various social and cultural factors. These alternative perspectives are described in Chapter 2. We also invited a presentation giving a historical overview of societal attitudes toward the retarded, from which the historical material in Chapter 2 is drawn.

This meeting included a discussion of various behavioral characteristics of the retarded that distinguish them from normal people. Most members of the group argued that while much behavior will overlap with that of normal people, nevertheless differences are sufficiently marked in retarded people to justify a delineation of that population. Others argued that whatever differences may exist do not warrant adopting any measures that may stigmatize the mentally retarded. Concerns over who gets labeled as "retarded" and where and when such labeling takes place followed from these various positions. The disagreements that arose over the benefits versus the liabilities of labeling the retarded are captured in Chapter 3.

Finally, in anticipation of the case study we had chosen to explore in the second half of the project, we included a talk on the legal dimensions of intervention with the retarded, using the example of involuntary sterilization. The two outcomes of protection of society versus benefit or harm to the retarded individual were contrasted. Discussion centered on the issues of paternalism and autonomy: Does the state have the right to act paternalistically (what is known in law as the *parens patriae* power) when it judges intervention to be on behalf of the retarded? Or should the autonomy of the individual be preserved even at the expense of his making serious mistakes (as one participant put it, "the right to fail")? The question of whether the mildly mentally retarded are capable of granting voluntary and informed consent was explored. These issues appear throughout Part I, but especially in Chapters 4, 6, and 7.

In the case study on sterilization of the retarded, we concentrated on two related topics: competence to be a good parent, and theoretical issues of voluntary and involuntary sterilization. We attempted to define the minimal requirements to be a good parent. Different kinds of criteria were introduced for assessing competence to raise children. Discussion among the group compared the proposed criteria with the minimal requirements that would *preclude* someone from being able to raise children. The issue of competence to raise children is taken up in Chapter 6.

We then introduced the question of sterilization of the retarded, both voluntary and involuntary, and asked when, if ever, these interventions are justified. Regarding voluntary sterilization, some of the key issues raised were whether the retarded are able to give voluntary and informed consent for such a procedure, whether third-party consent is properly construed as voluntary or involuntary, and what kind of stance should be taken in counseling the retarded—a paternalistic one, or a nondirective one that lets the retarded individual take his own risks. Discussion focused on the notion of "best interest" and which alternative is in the best interest of the mildly mentally retarded person—involuntary sterilization, or having a child one cannot take care of. A systematic presentation of the ethical and legal issues appears in Chapters 6 and 7.

Finally, we addressed ourselves to a discussion of several key legal cases that concerned sterilization of the retarded, joined with an overview of the legal history and trends in the law regarding sterilization. Chapter 5 presents these legal materials in some detail, and the Appendix to this volume includes excerpts from several key court cases. Although not all readers will be interested in the details of state statutes and judicial precedents, many should find the reasoning of the judges illuminating. In some instances the court addressed the ethical issues directly, placing them in the appropriate legal context. In others, however, moral concerns are subordinated to the exigencies of the law.

The format of this book requires a word of explanation. Part I is written as a narrative account, intended to convey the many conceptual, theoretical, moral, and legal issues that surround care and treatment of the mildly mentally retarded. Presented here as the outcome of a year's deliberations by an interdisciplinary group of scholars, it is written with the expectation that readers from many different disciplinary and theoretical perspectives will find this narrative approach a fruitful way of exploring the range of issues the project addressed. At the same time, we realize that readers interested in particular aspects of our study might want to have a fuller presentation of the key issues and arguments than the narrative format allows. We have, therefore, selected a number of the formal papers prepared by project participants for inclusion in Part II. This enables readers seeking well-developed philosophical arguments for or against various positions to study those arguments in greater detail. Although Part II does not offer a fully comprehensive background for the issues discussed in Part I, it should nonetheless provide readers with more in the way of ethical reasoning about these crucial concerns than is usually found in books devoted to the subject of mental retardation.

RUTH MACKLIN
WILLARD GAYLIN

Contents

Introduction

Each society has its own values and models of desirable behavior. Deviations from the culturally approved patterns are the basis for negative sanction, and, if serious enough, they can lead to isolation, confinement, and extermination. In a highly technological and economically competitive society such as ours, great value has been placed on intelligence, and persons whose intellectual skills are obviously less developed than the norm have traditionally been devalued and treated as deviants.

Special labels have been applied to such persons, and the labels have typically assumed highly derogatory connotations. Thus, such terms as "moron," "imbecile," and "idiot," although initially designed as scientific labels for special levels of mental retardation, have long since degenerated into general, colloquial put-downs. Even clinicians and scientists have, until quite recently, tended to equate low intelligence with poor prognosis and unresponsiveness to treatment. Hence, a label of mental retardation or its equivalent has tended to generate self-fulfilling and self-limiting prophecies.

This scientific hopelessness regarding retarded people can be related to two major elements. First, decreased intelligence has traditionally been interpreted as the result of defective development, injury, or disease of the brain. Since, until very recently, it was widely believed that brain tissue cannot repair itself nor be stimulated to develop, mental retardation and other conditions resulting from impaired brain development were defined as "irreversible" conditions. Second, the strong domination of psychiatry in the field of mental disabilities of all types until recently has had a generally stifling effect on the field of mental retardation. Strongly influenced by the psychoanalytic movement, psychiatry emphasized treatment approaches dependent on intellectual skills, including a highly developed ability to introspect, abstract, verbalize, and learn through insight. Therefore, retarded people were, often by definition, considered as unsuitable for psychiatric treatment or any form of psychotherapy. The only "treatment of choice" was custodial care, often accompanied by massive medication designed to control objectionable behavior.

A general hopelessness and pessimism permeated the professional community; and public opinion toward mental retardation was, until very recently, likewise predicated on negative stereotypes of retarded people. Wolfensberger (1969) has described several of these common popular models and their negative consequences for retarded persons. Thus, he describes the "Diseased Organism," the "Menace," the "Eternal Child," the "Object of Pity," the "Holy Infant," and the "Subhuman Organism." Each of these stereotypes leads to misunderstanding and mistaken evaluation of the retarded person.

The fundamental premise underlying society's general rejection of the mentally retarded is the implicit assumption that there are degrees of humanness, and that retarded people are not fully human. This assumption has provided the rationale justifying gross violations of human and legal rights, including infringement on fundamental constitutional rights. Indeed, it has repeatedly been clearly documented that many retarded persons have been subjected to indefinite confinement, cruel and unusual punishment, life-threatening human experimentation, and other forms of abuse. Chief among these has been the practice of involuntary sterilization, in the absence of procedural safeguards to protect the rights of the retarded.

The past two decades have witnessed dramatic changes in the field of mental retardation. The hopelessness which permeated the field during the first half of the century is being gradually replaced by positive and optimistic expectations.

Perhaps the most fundamental change has been the adoption of a developmental model of mental retardation, in contrast to the negative stereotypes identified by Wolfensberger. According to this model, every mentally retarded person is approached with the positive expectation that he has the potential to grow, develop, and learn. Emphasis is placed on the importance of environmental influences and the malleability of the organism. Hence, efforts are directed toward providing retarded individuals with conditions which foster their development. Specific developmental goals have been defined as "(1) increasing the complexity of behavior, (2) improving capacity to cope with the environment, and (3) enhancing human qualities" (as culturally defined) (Roos, 1972, p. 1065).

Another concept which has had major impact on the field of mental retardation is commonly referred to as normalization. Predicated on the recognition that deviancy in handicapped people has been fostered by differential treatment, labeling, and segregation, this principle advocates providing retarded persons with conditions which are as much like normal conditions as possible to foster culturally normative behavior. This approach is now widely applied to the delivery of services as well as to settings in which retarded persons live. The concept of educational mainstreaming, which is discussed at length in a subsequent chapter, is a specific application of this more general principle.

Emphasis on the variability among retarded people has been underlined by the principle of individualization, defined as "the recognition of the uniqueness of each handicapped person," resulting in "increasing emphasis on the individual program plan, on prescriptive programming, on the recognition that we must avoid regimentation" (Roos, 1975, p. 27). Hence, it is now generally accepted that applying uniform labels to such highly heterogeneous groups as mentally retarded people tends to reduce them to the least common denominator and to seriously interfere with individual growth and development. This principle has recently been incorporated in program guidelines, national standards for evaluating services, court decisions, and federal laws.

Another major principle now generally accepted in the field of mental retardation is the concept that every retarded person should be given maximum opportunity to determine his own course to shape his own destiny. Concretely applied, this principle means that whenever possible, the retarded person must be allowed the right to choose among alternative courses of action; that is, he must be granted freedom to the greatest extent possible. Indeed, the concept of least restrictive alternative, which underlies much of the recent class-action litigation on behalf of retarded persons, can be interpreted as that alternative which provides for greatest individual freedom (Roos, 1979).

The application of these basic principles is having major consequences for mentally retarded people. The field of mental retardation is currently in turmoil, with traditional approaches being replaced by emerging concepts. For example, as described in greater detail in a subsequent portion of this book, the medical model, long considered the most appropriate approach to mental retardation, is being replaced by multidisciplinary models emphasizing psychoeducational approaches. Likewise, large, multipurpose residential institutions as the backbone of services for retarded people are rapidly being replaced by community based, dispersed, small residential settings.

These dramatic changes have not occurred spontaneously. Rather, they are the outcome of complex forces which have shaped the development of services for retarded people during the past three decades. Some of the more obvious elements involved in fostering these changes include the following:

- Our society has been gradually shifting from a preoccupation with economic values toward greater concern with humanistic values. Inherent in this trend has been increasing emphasis on individual dignity and worth, including greater tolerance for deviancy from cultural norms.
- The civil rights movement has had important implications for many disenfranchised populations, including handicapped persons. As members of a minority group whose legal rights have traditionally been violated, retarded people have benefited from the legal and social reforms generated by civil rights activists, including court decisions and enactment of laws.
- Consumerism has likewise had an impact on mentally retarded people and their families. Indeed, parents of retarded people began to join together as early as the 1930s to improve the lot of their children. The founding of what is now the National Association for Retarded Citizens (NARC) in 1950 heralded a major step in improving conditions for retarded individuals. The NARC has played a key role in catalyzing changes in the field of mental retardation, relying primarily on activities in the areas of public education, legislation, and establishment of policies and national prototypes. More recently, the association has assumed a leadership role in mounting class-action suits resulting in precedent-setting court decisions.
- The personal interest in mental retardation of President Kennedy led him to initiate a number of federal efforts which fostered significant escalation in legislation as well as increased public understanding and support.

- Federal and state legislation has favored improved services to retarded people, in terms both of providing greatly expanded funding and establishing new programs and services.
- Class-action suits dealing with rights of retarded people have had major impact on services. The principal focuses of these cases have been right to treatment (e.g., *Pennsylvania Association for Retarded Children* v. *Pennsylvania; Mills* v. *Board of Education of the District of Columbia*) and improvement of institutional conditions (e.g., *Wyatt* v. *Stickney; New York State Association for Retarded Children* v. *Carey; Welsh* v. *Likins*).
- Improvement in technology appropriate to the habilitation and education of retarded people has helped to change professional indifference and hopelessness into enthusiastic optimism. Techniques based on behavior modification have been particularly useful in that they are applicable to nonverbal persons with very limited intelligence. Thus, the traditional assumption that retarded persons are unsuitable candidates for psychological approaches has been laid to rest.

This summary is by no means inclusive, but it illustrates the complexity of factors responsible for current changes in the field of mental retardation. The result has been improved services and a better quality of life for many retarded people. The gross abuse and neglect which were prevalent as recently as ten years ago are much reduced. Yet violations of rights still continue, many retarded individuals do not yet have access to appropriate services, and today's technology is still in its infancy. It would be naïve, therefore, to conclude that the needs of retarded people are now being fully met.

As basic legal rights of retarded people have gradually been recognized, and as improved technology has been applied to the problems of mental retardation, new and complex issues have begun to surface. Whereas the earlier issues relating to access to education and quality of institutional care were basically noncontroversial, these new issues have tended to generate considerable conflict. Often consumer advocates, mental retardation professionals, and interested members of the legal profession increasingly find themselves in disagreement on these emerging issues. All agree that they seek what is "best" for retarded people, but it is becoming less clear as to how to define "best." This difficulty is partly a function of the growing potency of technology which provides increasingly effective tools for controlling human beings and their future. Thus, many of the questions raised with regard to retarded people are merely specific instances of more general issues affecting all human beings. Examples include the application of genetic engineering, psychotechnology, and heroic approaches to preservation of life. Other issues are more specifically related to mental retardation in that they stem from concerns regarding the degree to which individual rights and privileges should be mitigated by decreased capacity. Examples of these types of issues include marriage, parenthood, and participation in human experimentation.

These types of issues obviously transcend the field of mental retardation—they strike at the very essence of the human condition. Likewise they are not the sole province of any single professional discipline, but they are relevant to philosophy, law, medicine, the behavioral sciences, and other professions. As our technology continues to expand, leading to ever-increasing control over our own destiny, we will experience growing urgency in resolving these types of issues.

It is against this background that we consider sterilization of mentally retarded people, as a specific instance illustrative of the types of issues just described. As retarded people increasingly join the mainstream of society as fully participating citizens, questions of marriage and child rearing are becoming commonplace. Hence analysis of the factors involved in sterilization is very germane to the field of mental retardation. Yet the fundamental ethical and legal issues transcend the specific situation of retarded people, for they relate to matters of individual freedom, capacity to choose, and the degree to which the individual controls his own destiny.

In the following chapters mental retardation is defined in terms of current developments in the field, and historical background is provided regarding educational services for retarded people. Problems related to labeling and the segregation–integration issue are selected for specific attention.

The matter of competence as it relates to mental retardation is explored in depth, followed by a presentation of the legal background related to sterilization of retarded people. The remaining chapters present detailed legal, ethical, and psychosocial aspects of this issue. No attempt is made to reach a consensus, but rather the various positions which surfaced among the members of the study group are presented, including legal, ethical, and scientific considerations. The deliberation of the participants concludes Part I with a summary of the group's speculations about the future.

PHILIP ROOS, PH.D.

REFERENCES

Mills v. *Board of Education of the District of Columbia*, 348 F. Supp. 866 (D.D.C., 1972).

New York State Association for Retarded Children v. *Carey*, 393 F. Supp. 715 (E.D., N.Y., 1975).

Pennsylvania Association for Retarded Children v. *Pennsylvania*, 343 F. Supp. 279 (E.D., Pa., 1972).

Roos, P., "Mentally Retarded Citizens: Challenge for the 1970's." *23 Syracuse Law Review* 1972: 1059

Roos, P., "Identification of Service-Related Research Needs in the Education of the Severely Handicapped." In *Proceedings of the Conference on Research Needs Related to Education of the Severely Handicapped*. Washington, D.C.: Bureau of Education for the Handicapped, U.S. Office of Education (1975), pp. 25–35.

Roos, P., "The Law and Mentally Retarded People: An Uncertain Future." *Stanford Law Review*, 31(4), April, 1979.

Welsch v. *Likins*, 343 F. Supp. 485 (U. S. D. Ct., Minn., 1974).
Wolfensberger, W., "The Origin and Nature of Our Institutional Models," in: *Changing Patterns in Residential Services for the Mentally Retarded*, eds. R. B. Kugel & W. Wolfensberger, pp. 59–1716. (Washington, D.C.: President's Committee on Mental Retardation (1969).
Wyatt v. *Stickney*, 344 F. Supp. 387 (M. D. Ala., 1972), aff'd sub. nom. *Wyatt* v. *Aderholt* 503 F. 2d 1305 (5th Cir. 1974).

PART I

CHAPTER I

An Awareness of Consequences

We live in a time marked by proliferating demands for civil rights, economic rights, human rights, and individual rights as expressed by an extremely diverse number of groups who believe themselves to be discriminated against in our society and who regard themselves in one way or another as "minorities." These groups can be quite small or very large. The physically handicapped—in particular those confined to wheelchairs—are a relatively small group that has launched an increasingly effective campaign demanding that both the public and private sector provide ramps and other amenities that will facilitate their ability to live as normally as possible. The elderly, proclaiming "gray rights," have successfully influenced Congress to extend the mandatory-retirement age to 70, a change in the law that will affect many millions of people.

Yet, because we live in a pluralistic society, the extension of rights in one area is often seen as an infringement on the rights of others. Thus as soon as one group begins to achieve success in effecting the changes they desire, other new groups spring up to counter such changes. Antibusing groups oppose desegregation decisions on the grounds that the rights of their children to go to neighborhood schools are being abrogated. Feminist support for the Equal Rights Amendment has resulted in the formation of counter groups anxious to preserve what they see as traditional prerogatives and exemptions for women. The gay rights movement has been challenged by a vociferous campaign to prevent homosexuals from being employed as teachers. Such debates are given enormous media coverage, with the conflicting claims being sorted out in court cases, plebiscites, and through executive orders on the local, state, and national levels. Since the results of such actions vary widely in different parts of the country, most of these conflicts remain unsettled.

It is against this background that we are here considering the situation of a minority group that has been largely unable to organize on its own either to define or to press for its rights. This group is the mildly mentally retarded. Some conferences of mentally retarded persons have taken place in the United States, Canada, England, and Sweden, but these efforts have not as yet attained the scope or impact of the national organizations of other minority groups. Despite the adoption of a declaration of the rights of the mentally handicapped by the United Nations General Assembly in 1971, and the endorsement of this declaration by the President's Committee on Mental Retardation, the rights of the retarded continue to be restricted in many states. We will be examining the arguments on which such restrictions are based, exploring the psychological, social, and ethical aspects of the problem. Our particular emphasis will be on the question of whether or not the mentally retarded should have the right to marry and bear children, and whether the granting of these rights constitutes a benefit or a burden for the retarded. These questions will be viewed in the context of a number of court cases involving voluntary or involuntary sterilization of the mildly retarded.

In order to put the question of sterilization in proper perspective, we will also be dealing with the criteria by which mental retardation is defined, alternative forms of education and treatment, and the ability of the mildly retarded to function competently in a variety of societal situations. A consideration of the rights of the mentally retarded raises fundamental questions about the relationship between societal responsibility and human freedom, and thus can serve to illuminate the problems involved in determining the rights of many other groups seeking to extend (or retain) their own rights.

Although disagreements as to terminology exist, the mentally retarded are often divided into four different categories, reflecting increasing levels of retardation. The least affected are the *mildly retarded,* followed by the *moderately retarded,* the *severely retarded,* and the *profoundly retarded.* It is perhaps more useful, however, to describe the retarded in terms of their *educability.* Those in the mildly retarded group are often educable to a considerable extent, are basically able to care for themselves, and to function adequately in a number of societal situations. The more severely retarded show correspondingly less ability in all these areas, with the profoundly retarded unable to care for most of their basic needs. It should be noted that a number of experts in the field of mental retardation believe that with new approaches in teaching methods and more sophisticated technology, it will be possible in the future to help greater numbers of even the profoundly retarded to learn to care for themselves more adequately. This, however, is only one point of view, and the potential educability of the retarded remains a highly volatile question to which we will be addressing considerable attention.

In recent years, the number of retarded persons living in institutions has decreased considerably. Most mildly retarded persons live in society, whether alone, with relatives, or with other mildly retarded individuals. In this study we have concentrated on the mildly retarded not only because they comprise the vast majority of retarded persons, but also because the distinctions between mildly retarded and "normal" individuals are often blurred. In fact, several members of our research group were unwilling to draw a hard line between the mildly retarded and normal persons. Others of us feel that such a line can be drawn, but the very fact that disagreement exists on this crucial question gives it special pertinence. It is exactly because the mildly retarded exist on the borderline between low-normal intelligence and the more severely retarded that ethical and legal difficulties arise in determining their rights. Throughout this book, references to the "retarded" can be taken to mean the *mildly* retarded unless otherwise specified.

In many states the mildly retarded, even though they are not institutionalized, must submit to the guidance of other persons or authorities before making key life decisions—including the decision to marry, to have children, to enter into financial contracts, and to live alone. Indeed, the term "guidance" is not strictly accurate in describing the relationship of a legally incompetent person and his or her legal guardian. Technically, the retarded person is often denied the right to make such decisions at all—contracts made by the retarded are void, marriages may be annulled, and so on. Thus adults of normal intelligence may often make these decisions for the retarded without getting the consent of anyone at all, although, as we shall see, this situation has changed in some states as the result of court decisions.

In court cases involving the retarded, the central issue is usually the retarded person's *competence* or lack of it. From a legal standpoint, competence essentially refers to the process of acquiring knowledge, the ability to select and express one's choices, and the ability to decide rationally. The legal tradition has been to classify people on this basis as either competent or incompetent. Yet questions arise as to whether such distinctions are valid. Although there are obvious extremes of competence and incompetence, many cases in which legal determinations are made fall in between such extremes. In such instances, therefore, some would claim that competence can be meaningfully defined only with relevance to a specific situation. That is, an individual may be competent in respect to one situation and incompetent in respect to another.

The willingness of the court to find partial competence in some areas while acknowledging incompetence in others is a fairly recent development. Previously, competence was seen as an "all-or-none" phenomenon.[1] The determination of partial competence calls into question, of course, the usefulness and relevance of standard IQ measurements and classification procedures. What is the relationship between an IQ of 70 and the ability to decide one's own goals and means of attaining them? What correspondences are there between an understanding of intellectual abstractions and the ability to function in society? Are, perhaps, standard tests in themselves an unfair way of determining the capacities of the retarded?

The answers to such questions are of importance not only in respect to legal determinations but in respect to how the mentally retarded are to be treated in general. They affect, for instance, the issue of the kind of education that those identified as mentally retarded should receive. There are two major schools of thought concerning this issue, and proponents of both schools participated in our research group. One school believes that the mildly retarded, for their own benefit, should be educated separately from normal children. The other school holds that the retarded have a greater opportunity to fulfill their potential if they are "mainstreamed," educated in classes with normal children. Here again, the fundamental question of the rights of the retarded emerges. Is the right of the mentally retarded person to be protected from harm of greater importance than his or her right to live as normally as possible? Are retarded persons who are edu-

[1]For further discussion of the legal traditions regarding definitions of competence, see Chapter 11.

cated together with normal children more likely to develop competence in a greater number of areas, or, on the contrary, does "mainstreaming" expose them to an increased danger of being exploited or victimized?

A consideration of these questions is complicated by the fact that the symptoms of mental retardation may be observed in persons who differ vastly in behavior and competence. Some retarded children experience few difficulties in living at home and attending regular school classes, while others present such severe management problems that placement in a highly structured residential program is sometimes required. Many persons with mental retardation demonstrate learning problems that show up only in academic pursuits; yet others are so impaired that the acquisition of basic self-care skills involves considerable effort. Diversity is also apparent in the causes of mental retardation. Diminished intellectual function can arise from a host of single or interacting factors: gene defects, chromosomal aberrations, inheritance of inferior polygenes, central nervous system trauma, and psychosocial deprivation.

It seems clear that as this diversity of causative factors and these variations in behavioral competence have become more widely recognized, they have influenced the courts to move away from the sweeping "all-or-none" decisions of the past, and instead to base judgments on partial competence in specific areas. Yet even in making more narrowly based judgments, the courts have been extremely inconsistent in a number of cases involving the sterilization of the mentally retarded. It could hardly be otherwise, since different states have widely divergent laws pertaining to the rights of the mentally retarded. These variations in the law may result in the performance of unwarranted sterilization in one locality while in another locality sterilizations that seem more clearly warranted may be ruled out.

In a later chapter we will be discussing these court cases in detail as a background to the broader consideration of the ethical issues involved in the sterilization of the mentally retarded. The court cases themselves often focus on the question of whether or not the particular individual is competent to raise a child, but there are larger questions that must be addressed. For example, it can be argued that since many of the mildly retarded have normal sexual needs, it is to their own benefit to voluntarily submit to sterilization, in that they will then be free to express their sexuality without concern that they may produce children for whom they could not properly care. But from another point of view it can be argued that sterilization robs the retarded of the basic human right to bear children. We will be dealing with the ethics of involuntary sterilization, as well as discussing whether or not the retarded are capable of making a decision, with full awareness of its consequences, to undergo voluntary sterilization.

The concept of an "awareness of consequences" has been a recurrent theme throughout the course of this study. It is a concept that has relevance to determining the criteria by which the retarded may be identified; it figures largely in the question of whether or not a line can be drawn between the mildly retarded and persons of normal intelligence; and it has an important bearing on the debate as to whether the retarded should be educated separately or in regular classes with normal children. And it is fundamental to making a determination of competence or incompetence.

Throughout our deliberations, moreover, the members of this research group have been acutely concerned with analyzing the consequences and implications of our various points of view concerning the rights and needs of the retarded. Because our points of view *are* various, our aim in this book is not to provide final answers, but rather to illuminate the complexity of the issues involved. In the course of our work, some potential options for the future have suggested themselves, but our chief concern is to clarify the differences of philosophical approach and practical application that exist among the members of this research group and in society at large. Only by grasping the essence of these differences and understanding the reasons for them can a coherent approach to the rights of the mildly retarded eventually be arrived at. Thus this book is in essence a debate. Contrasting views will be set against one another, not with the intention of providing a "winner," but rather with the purpose of delineating *all* viewpoints as clearly as possible. We disagree on many things, but we are emphatically in accord on the importance of the debate itself.

In the past, the retarded have too often been seen as "separate" from the rest of humanity. This kind of stigmatization has of course affected other minority groups. Thus, in the course of our debate, we hope to be able to make a contribution to the overall question within the context of a pluralistic society of the rights of individuals, minorities, or special groups. The responsibility of a society to maintain the common good will inevitably come into conflict at times with the rights of individual members of that society. In attempting to achieve a balance between the common good and individual rights, the greater awareness we have of the particular problems and aspirations of special groups, the greater is our potential for coming to grips, wisely and fairly, with the inherent difficulties of the democratic ideal.

CHAPTER 2

Toward a Definition of Mental Retardation

Historically, the ways in which the mentally retarded have been viewed and treated has often been a reflection of the dominant spirit of the times within a particular culture.[1] But whether retarded individuals were ignored, ridiculed, incarcerated, cast out, or looked upon with beneficence, attempts to comprehend and define the phenomena of retardation were few and far between until fairly recent times.

Although the ancient Greeks were the first to make written reference to the retarded, their understanding of the condition did not go much beyond acknowledging its existence. Because of the profound emphasis that the Greeks placed upon form, symmetry, and beauty, children who were born with physical deformities or who were recognized as "defective" were put to death. In addition, anatomical dissection

[1]The historical material in this and other chapters is drawn in part from an audiovisual production prepared by Dr. Charles Keramidas for the Georgia Retardation Center.

was forbidden even on those so destroyed, effectively inhibiting scientific inquiry. Many of the infants that were put to death were very likely not at all mentally retarded, but simply physically malformed. Those individuals who were recognized as retarded after infancy survived only if they proved useful, usually in the capacity of a slave or servant. Others, as described by Plato, were left in a "strange and unknown place" to die. In 500 B.C. Hippocrates described certain deformities of the skull characteristic of some severe types of mental retardation, but in general the Greek emphasis on physical form confused the issue, and little attempt was made to classify the retarded in terms of mental ability.

In the East, a more benign attitude toward the retarded was taken. At about the same period that Hippocrates was writing, Zoroaster (400 B.C.) and Confucius (500 B.C.) were advocating "tender care" of all those recognized as "different," a sentiment that was not voiced in the Western world for nearly a thousand years. But in the East as well as in the West, there was no real investigation of the mentally retarded that might lead to any form of definition or classification.

Over the next fifteen hundred years considerable changes occurred regarding the ways in which the mentally retarded were dealt with, and these will be discussed in the succeeding chapter on the subject of treatment and education of the retarded. In terms of developing a definition of the retarded, however, these many centuries brought little progress. The mentally retarded and the mentally insane were generally lumped together in the same category. It was not until the sixteenth and seventeenth centuries that this situation began to change. Fitz-Herbert promulgated a legal definition of idiocy in 1534. In 1675 Hoefer delivered the first scientific treatise on cretinism. Such terms as "idiocy" and "cretinism" reflect the fact that the distinctions being made were still crude ones, however.

Thomas Willis included a chapter on mental retardation in his medical text, published in 1672. On the subject of classification, he noted that among the retarded "some are unable to learn their letters but can handle mechanical arts; others who fail at this can easily comprehend agriculture; others are unfit except to eat and sleep; others merely dolts or driveling fools."

John Locke, who, in 1690, was the first to distinguish idiocy from insanity, had a great effect upon the development of a concept of mental retardation. He popularized the idea that the intellect was only a storehouse for information gathered by the senses. In distinguishing between the retarded and the insane, he said that the insane put together wrong ideas while the retarded put forth no ideas. Locke's theories, as we shall see, had considerable influence on both the treatment and education of the retarded. But the next major steps in terms of classification did not come until the early nineteenth century. Jean Esquirol, the French psychiatric pioneer, who was among the first to recognize the emotional basis of mental disorders, also stated that idiocy was not a disease but a condition originating at the beginning of life. He proposed two separate levels of mental retardation—idiocy and imbecility—with the differentiation between the two being made on the basis of differences in speech capacity.

In the late nineteenth century, a new direction was taken when medical as opposed to psychological criteria began to be developed. In 1866 Langdon Down described mongolism—which is now referred to as Down's syndrome. His use of the term "mongolism" was derived from facial appearance and based upon a theory of regression to alleged lower races. Down later turned away from the racial theory, and went on to develop the first extended medical classification system. The first component of this system was congenital idiocy, encompassing both microcephaly, marked by an extremely small skull that does not allow room for proper development of the brain, and hydrocephaly, a condition in which excess fluid causes great enlargement of the skull and corresponding pressure upon the brain. In the congenital category, Down also included paralysis and epilepsy. The second component of this system focused on developmental idiocy, which Down ascribed to anxiety in reaction to cutting teeth and the onset of puberty; this classification, informed more by Victorian prejudice than by scientific analysis, was later discredited. Down also included a category for accidental injury or illness leading to brain damage, but it is his work on congenital retardation that survives as his most important contribution to the field.

Other medical researchers soon described syphilitic retardation, tuberous sclerosis, and Tay-Sachs disease. These and subsequent identifications of specific genetic and biological syndromes caused a shift of emphasis in research on the mentally retarded. The specificity of medical definitions and criteria made them easier to deal with than psychological ones, and the *medical model* of mental retardation became dominant for a considerable period. But the medical model left many unanswered questions. The medical model was useful in identifying organic causes of retardation, particularly among the severely and profoundly retarded. But the vast majority of the mildly retarded, and many of the moderately retarded, do not suffer from any identifiable medical syndrome.

Today, therefore, although the medical model remains a pertinent diagnostic tool in respect to certain types of retardation, the emphasis has changed once again, with psychological and sociological factors being given the greatest attention. Indeed, these factors are increasingly considered even in the case of the small minority of retarded individuals in whom a specific organic cause can be identified.

Because of the heterogeneous factors that are now recognized as playing a part in the causation of mental retardation, no single explanatory scheme can be expected to fully explain the phenomenon. The fact that there can be considerable *behavioral* differences between individuals with similar IQ scores and similar social backgrounds further complicates efforts to develop a consistent theoretical approach. Nevertheless, there are various approaches that can be useful in clarifying at least some aspects of the problem. One such framework is the cognitive-developmental perspective, as presented principally in the work of Zigler,[2] and elaborated by a number of investigators of the developmental psychology of the mentally retarded child. This perspective is aligned with the theories of normal child development espoused by Piaget.[3]

The basic tenet of the Ziglerian point of view is that the largest single diagnostic group of the mentally retarded is composed of individuals whose cognitive competencies, as measured by standard IQ tests, are similar to those of younger nonretarded persons. Thus, in terms of the hierarchy of intellectual stages of development established by Piaget and others, the mentally retarded are hypothesized to develop intellectual skills at a slower rate than nonretarded persons; moreover, it is assumed that their ultimate level of intellectual achievement corresponds to a developmental plateau that the nonretarded progress beyond.

The use of IQ tests to measure the cognitive abilities of the retarded is widespread but controversial. Some members

[2]This presentation of Zigler's theories is based upon five separate publications: E. Zigler, "Mental Retardation: Current Issues and Approaches," in L. W. Hoffman and M. L. Hoffman, eds., *Review of Child Development Research*, vol. 2 (New York: Russell Sage Foundation, 1966); E. Zigler, "Familial Mental Retardation: A Continuing Dilemma," *Science* 155 (1967): 292–298; E. Zigler, "Developmental versus Difference: Theories in Mental Retardation and the Problem of Motivation," *American Journal of Mental Deficiency* 73 (1969): 536–556; E. Zigler, "The Retarded Child as a Whole Person," in D. K. Routh, ed., *The Experimental Psychology of Mental Retardation* (Chicago: Aldine, 1973); E. Zigler, "Research on Personality Structure in the Retardate," in N. R. Ellis, ed., *International Review of Research in Mental Retardation*, vol. 1 (New York: Academic Press, 1966).

[3]The following books and articles by Piaget are of particular importance in the context of mental retardation: B. Inhelder and J. Piaget, *The Growth of Logical Thinking from Childhood to Adolescence* (New York: Basic Books, 1958); J. Piaget, and B. Inhelder, *The Psychology of the Child* (New York: Basic Books, 1969); J. Piaget, "Intellectual Evolution from Adolescence to Adulthood," *Human Development* 15 (1972): 1–12; J. Piaget, "Preface" in B. Inhelder, *Diagnosis of Reasoning in the Mentally Retarded, 1st ed.* (New York: John Day, 1968).

of our research group questioned the significance of certain levels of scoring in differentiating the mildly retarded from the "normal" person, while others doubted the validity of using the tests at all. But let us leave aside these questions for the moment. The debate concerning the use of IQ tests can be more clearly understood if we first examine Piaget's theories of childhood development and Zigler's application of these theories to the cognitive abilities of the retarded.

Piaget and his colleagues have postulated the existence of several universal major periods and stages of cognitive growth. The first period, characterizing the cognitive activity of the infant, is termed the *sensorimotor* period. There is no need to discuss this stage here, since it is obvious that all mildly retarded persons pass through and beyond this stage to achieve higher levels of cognitive sophistication. The second major period covers early and middle childhood in intellectually normal persons and is divided into stages, the first consisting of *preoperational thought* and the second of *concrete operational thought*.

In the preoperational stage of this developmental period, thought becomes symbolic but is characterized by a number of structural features which are as yet unable to provide the person with an information-processing system that is both stable and efficient. At this level a number of frequently observed characteristics of prelogical thought are evident. The child's thought processes are static and inflexible, marked by distortions caused by the failure to consider multiple perspectives. The child reasons transductively, from the specific to the specific rather than from the specific to the general. Instead of forming concepts by mentally combining a number of particulars, the thought processes are dominated by precepts—the child will be quiet while a parent is talking on the telephone because the parent has told him to stop talking, not because he understands that it is impossible to listen to two conversations at once. Such cognitive operations as classification, seriation, and conservation are still deficient; for instance, because both a cat and a cloud move, the child will classify both as being alive; the child will be able to arrange colored blocks in a series, but not ideas; and the child is not yet able to comprehend that when water is poured from a container of one shape into a container of a different shape the mass of the water has been conserved and is the same. This list of cognitive limitations details an egocentric mental structure that is still poorly equipped for competent problem solving and sophisticated reasoning and judgment.

However, in the intellectually average child, the appearance of concrete operational thought is observed at about the age of seven. This second stage of development in the early and middle childhood period is marked by greater efficiency in a number of critical respects, and leads to the emergence of a stable information-processing system and the appearance of logical problem-solving strategies. Equipped with these competencies, the child is able to adapt to additional features of both the physical and the social-interpersonal world. These new capabilities are shown by the ability to maintain conceptual stability amid the flux of perceived events, and in the use of deliberate as well as covert mental strategies to assist both memorial and problem-solving skills. They are also revealed in the establishment and maintenance of cooperative and reciprocal interactions with others, in a fledgling appreciation of the phenomenology of others as separate entities, and in an emergent organization of values, social rules, and the responsibilities such rules entail.

The final stage in the Piagetian hierarchy is marked by the possession of formal operational thought. There are a number of ways in which formal thought differs from concrete operational thought. Concrete thought is limited to an awareness of concrete, "here-and-now" events and propositions. By comparison, formal thought proceeds from hypothesis and is deductive. A simple example can illustrate one difference between concrete operational and formal operational thought. A child—or a retarded adult—possessed of concrete operational thought would be able to take a subway or bus over a learned route between one destination and another. But if that subway or bus line was out of commission, an individual would need to have progressed to formal operational thought in order to devise by himself an alternate route and determine how much additional traveling time would be necessary to arrive at the destination on schedule.

The applications of formal thought, however, go far beyond the kind of mundane task exemplified by the above example. Formal thought directs action and behavior through reflection and introspection; the consequences of prior actions are considered and elaborated upon when taking new actions. Persons who have attained formal thought tend to consider a range of *available* alternatives in decision-making situations, and are able to make choices based on higher principles rather than simply on the basis of the immediate rewards or punishments of the moment. This capability does not guarantee, of course, that decisions will necessarily be made in terms of higher principles or future considerations, but the ability to take these aspects of the situation into account will at least be present. Obviously, formal thought is a necessary condition for the formulation of life plans as well as for the elaboration of means to reach life goals.

Let us now look at how this Piagetian hierarchy of development has been applied by Zigler and others to the mentally retarded. Such applications involve certain correlations between the stages outlined by Piaget and IQ test scores. When IQ scores are used in attempting to define mental retardation, it has been the practice to assign a cutoff point on a graph reflecting the usual distribution of IQ levels in the general population, with a mean score of 100. Currently, the line of demarcation is usually located at 70. Thus, in this system of classification, persons with a score of 70 or below are considered to be retarded.

In terms of the Piagetian hierarchy, then, the profoundly and severely retarded often do not progress significantly beyond the first stage, the sensorimotor period that characterizes the cognitive activity of infancy. Fundamentally unable to care for themselves, they are often institutionalized. What evidence is available indicates that most adults classified as moderately retarded by IQ—with scores ranging from 36 to 54—demonstrate the preoperational thinking that marks the first stage of Piaget's second major period.[4] Few, however, are found to have progressed to the next substage of this period, the level of concrete operations.

Available research suggests that most adults whose tested intelligence falls into the range of mild mental retardation—with scores from 54 to 70—do in fact acquire the cognitive competencies associated with the concrete operational level: the ability to maintain conceptual stability, the use of both deliberate and covert mental strategies in problem solving, and the establishment of reciprocal and cooperational interaction with others.

Thus, in terms of the Piagetian hierarchy, distinctions between the mildly retarded and those of "normal" intelligence must rest upon the presence or lack of formal operational thought, the final stage evidenced by the ability to structure content that is abstract, hypothetical, verbal, or involves the future. And here we encounter certain difficulties. Some investigators have presented evidence suggesting that a small portion of adults with IQs in the normal range do not demonstrate formal thought on Piagetian assessment tasks.[5]

[4]The available evidence concerning IQ scores and their correlation with preoperational thinking may be found in the following works: M. Woodward, "The Application of Piaget's Theory to Research in Mental Deficiency," in N. R. Ellis, ed., *Handbook of Mental Deficiency* (New York: McGraw-Hill, 1963); J. R. Kershner, "Conservation of Vertical-Horizontal Space Perception in Trainable Retarded Children," *American Journal of Mental Deficiency* 77 (1973): 710–716; K. Lovell, "The Developmental Approach of Jean Piaget," in M. Garrison, ed., "Cognitive Models and Development in Mental Retardation," *American Journal of Mental Deficiency* 70, (1966): 84–95; K. Wilton and F. J. Boersman, "Conservation Research with the Mentally Retarded," in N. R. Ellis, ed., *International Review of Research in Mental Retardation* vol. 7 (New York: Academic Press, 1974).

[5]For evidence concerning lack of formal thought in adults with normal IQ range, see: J. W. McKinnon and J. W. Renner, "Are Colleges Concerned with Intellectual Development?" *American Journal of Physics* 39 (1971): 1047–1052; M. Schwebel, "Formal Operations in First Year College Students," *Journal of Psychology* 91 (1975): 133–141.

Short-term training efforts are usually successful in leading nonretarded persons to apply formal structures to Piagetian problems, providing evidence that formal structural competence does exist in these persons. Such training efforts have not, however, been successful with persons who are mildly retarded. Therefore it is inferred that such individuals have not acquired formal thought structure.

But difficulties remain, and those who question the validity of IQ tests in distinguishing between the mildly retarded and the person of average intelligence are quick to point them out. Thus, short-term training efforts, as noted above, are *usually* but not *always* successful in assisting those who fail to demonstrate formal thought structures on assessment tasks. If a person of normal intelligence and a person of below-average intelligence both fail to demonstrate formal thought, might this not indicate the unreliability of IQ tests in certain cases? Does it not suggest a certain arbitrariness in drawing the line of demarcation between normality and retardation at the 70 scoring level? More important, does an IQ score of 69 necessarily mean that the individual is incapable of making decisions concerning the conduct of his or her own life in our society? Can a convincing case be made that a person with an IQ of 69 lacks certain crucial abilities that impair his or her functioning in job situations, family situations, or which make it necessary to withhold the right to having a bank account or voting? Does a person with an IQ 10 points higher possess these abilities in a sufficiently greater degree to classify the person as "normal?"

In order to fully confront these questions a distinction must first be made between two different kinds of mental retardation, based upon causative criteria. To begin with, we have the *medical model*. According to some estimates, about 25 percent of those classified as mentally retarded may be said to suffer from one or more of a variety of physiological defects, the existence of which is associated with their lower IQs. Among such defects are recessive-gene disorders, such as galactosemia and phenylketonuria; dominant-gene disorders such as tuberous sclerosis and neurofibromatosis; and chromosomal anamolies such as Down's syndrome. Some mentally retarded individuals may have suffered damage to their central nervous systems in either the prenatal or postnatal period, whether from prenatal infections, nutritional deficiencies affecting the fetus or the child after it is born, radiation, anoxia, head injury, or lead poisoning. Mentally retarded persons found to have been affected by any of these conditions may be said to be "defective" in a strict medical sense, since they possess some deficient physiological structure or experience some defective physiological process.

Yet it must be emphasized that the vast majority of persons who score below 70 on IQ tests do not qualify as defective by medical and neurophysiological criteria. These individuals, who constitute 90 percent of those classified as mildly retarded according to IQ scores (in the 55–69 range), belong rather to the second major group of the retarded, the "cultural-familial" or "undifferentiated" category.[6] Cultural-familial mental retardation is a presumptive rather than a positive diagnosis. In such cases there is a lack of evidence pointing to a cerebral pathological condition, but low intelligence may be found in other family members. This diagnosis is usually not made until school entry. Such children usually come from impoverished environments with poor housing, nutrition, and medical care.

The question of the causes of cultural-familial mental retardation remains one of the more controversial areas of debate among students of mental retardation. Whereas some writers have pointed to normal polygenic variation as an explanation of low intelligence without organic impairment, others have stressed the primary role of social and cultural factors leading to lower IQs in this group. Indeed it is in

[6]There is some disagreement as to the percentages of the retarded that should be classified in various categories. For support of the 90 percent figure cited here, see N. M. Robinson and H. B. Robinson, *The Mentally Retarded Child: A Psychological Approach* (New York: McGraw-Hill, 1976).

regard to this point that the most strenuous objections to the use of IQ tests in measuring the abilities of the mildly retarded are voiced.

Those who object to the use of standard psychological testing point out that within a homogeneous cultural setting the definition of abnormal behavior is a relatively straightforward task, because there is a general consensus as to what defines "normal" versus "aberrant" behavior. But within a culturally heterogeneous society, such as the United States, definitions of abnormality become increasingly problematic. Except for biologically damaged persons whose behavior would be regarded as abnormal in any human society, there may be profound differences of opinion concerning the nature of normality. Thus the identification of the mentally retarded through standard IQ tests and psychological assessment, faces both conceptual and technical difficulties in culturally diverse societies, according to this argument. And these difficulties become particularly acute in the assessment of organically intact persons who are not members of the cultural group that is dominant in the society. The fact that so many of the mildly retarded, whom we are focusing on here, come from impoverished environments accentuates the difficulty of accurate assessment.

In this argument, the United States is seen as an example of a culturally diverse society in which public policy has been based on a *conformity model*. The dominant group in the society for 300 years has been the English-speaking Caucasians. The language, institutions, history, values, and lifestyle of this dominant group are perpetuated through public education as a matter of public policy, with the goal of public education being to acculturate the children of minority groups to the language and culture of the dominant group and to wean them away from the language and culture of their parents. It is pointed out that assessment practices become part of the societal mechanism for enforcing and legitimating cultural conformity. Standardized tests, including IQ tests, are designed to predict success in the monolingual and monocultural public schools. Tests are written in the language of the dominant culture, and test content is specific to that culture. Consequently, a child from a nondominant minority is compared with children from the dominant group. Because he or she does not participate fully in the dominant culture, the average child from a minority group is likely to perform less well than a child being reared in the dominant cultural framework.[7]

Those who support standardized testing claim that the tests are valid because they accurately predict that children from minority backgrounds will perform less well academically. Some recent special programs have shown, however, that minority children show greater interest and aptitude when they are allowed to express themselves in terms consistent with their background. For instance, some researchers have attempted to show that there is a distinct "black" language, with its own consistent grammatical rules. This contention was tested in a number of schools, and it was found that when black children were asked to write essays in accepted textbook English, the results were imaginatively constricted and contained numerous errors in grammar and spelling. When they were given the opportunity to write on the same subject using the black idiom, the results were not only far more creative and expressive, but were marked by very few errors in terms of established linguistic usage among blacks. Such attempts to broaden the monolingual basis of public education have been attacked on the grounds that the future social and economic success of the children involved depends upon their learning to express themselves according to established standards. But such experiments have shown

[7]For further elucidation of the argument concerning the prediction, based upon IQ tests, that minority students will perform more poorly academically, see T. Cleary, L. G. Humphreys, S. A. Kendrick, and A. Wesman, *American Psychologist* 30 (1975): 15–41.

that when minority children are allowed to express themselves in the customary idiom of their families and neighbors, they produce results quite different from their usual work.

Whether or not such experimental teaching techniques are effective in preparing children to deal with our society, they raise an important point in respect to standardized testing. Because such tests based on the conformity model do not take into account variant forms of expression, they have, according to the views of some researchers restricted the educational opportunities of minority children by assigning disproportionately large numbers to classes for the mentally retarded.[8] In addition, the cultural-conformity model is seen as fostering a confusion between "prognosis" and "diagnosis." Tests designed as prognostic measures for predicting the future performance of the student have sometimes been interpreted as if they yield diagnostic information explaining the level of the child's performance—in other words, an IQ score of less than 70 may be accepted as *evidence* of mental retardation.

Those who support the use of IQ tests are not, however, unaware of these problems themselves. Although Zigler, for instance, makes use of IQ scores in his work, he has noted that:

> If one fails to appreciate the arbitrary nature of the 70 IQ cutoff point and the fact that we are dividing people on nothing more than the grossest overall measure of cognitive functioning, it is but a short step to the formulation that all those falling below this point compose a class of subnormals. Since the conceptual distance between "subnormal" and "abnormal"—the latter with its age old connotations of disease and defect—is minimal, the final easy step is to regard the retarded as a homogeneous group of organisms defective in all spheres of functioning and forever separate by their very nature from all persons possessing a higher IQ.

---

[8]In regard to the cultural-conformity model and the testing of minority children, see J. Mercer, *Labeling the Mentally Retarded: Clinical and Social Perspectives on Mental Retardation* (Berkeley: University of California Press, 1973).

The dangers inherent in the association between subnormality and abnormality can be mitigated by broadening the assessment basis. Some would argue that one of the fundamental steps that needs to be taken in this direction is to give full recognition to the pluralistic nature of our society. A view of society based on a *pluralistic model* is considerably more complex than one based on the *conformity model* previously discussed. The pluralistic view presents a culturally diverse society organized around a core culture consisting of the common language(s) and the basic political and economic institutions which hold society together. Various cultural groups, in this model, will have varying relationships to this core culture. In our society, for example, some groups have been both culturally and structurally absorbed—such as the German Protestants, the Scotch-Irish, and the Scandinavians. Other groups, although acculturated in many ways, still maintain sufficient structural separatism to remain identifiable. Irish Catholics and Jews would be examples of such groups in the United States. Other groups span the boundaries of the core culture. Some members of these groups may be recent migrants who do not speak the language of the core culture, and who may share only a minority of its values, beliefs, or ways of behaving.

When a pluralistic model of society forms the basis for developing an assessment system, conformity to the expectations of the monocultural school will not suffice as the basis for validating test instruments. Definitions of validity would need to be broadened to include performance in nonschool social roles. Test language and test content would have to be multilingual and multicultural. Rather than using a single norm, multiple normative frameworks would be necessary, so that an individual's performance could be compared not only with that of the core culture but also with the performance of others from a similar sociocultural background. Multicultural tests would, the proponents of the pluralistic model believe, make possible a clear separation of prognostic information which predicts role performance in a particular social system and diagnostic information which seeks to explain the cause of a particular performance.

Such an implementation of the pluralistic view for assessment purposes would, of course, involve basic changes in testing procedures, reflecting similar changes in the school curriculum itself—multilingual classes, for example. The practical obstacles to making such changes are considerable. In addition, there are those who feel that pluralistic assessment techniques could engender new problems and confusions about the retarded. For although the intent of pluralistic assessment proposals is to make certain that individuals are not labeled as retarded simply because they are not sufficiently acculturated in terms of the conformity model, a situation could be created in which still another label was being applied. That is, those found to be retarded through pluralistic assessment techniques would be labeled not merely retarded but "retarded Puerto Ricans" or "retarded blacks." Since one of the elements envisioned in a pluralistic school curriculum is multilingual teaching, the retarded might find themselves separated not only from "normal" children into special classes, but separated also from other retarded children according to their particular cultural background.

Thus, while the pluralistic model serves to remind us that current assessment techniques are far from perfect, some of us feel that it creates difficulties of its own. There are, however, aspects of the pluralistic model which, when combined with other assessment models, offer some possible options for the future, and we will return to these in a later chapter. Certainly it is true that unsuitable tests are particularly likely to be administered to those from minority groups, some of whom ought not to be considered retarded and for whom culture-bound IQ tests underestimate intellectual functions. But there are also other reasons why an individual who ought not to be classified as retarded may nevertheless exhibit a measured intelligence in the range of mild retardation. Many of these reasons are not related—or only indirectly related—to the cultural diversity of our society. A child of average mental ability from a culturally dominant background, for example, may simply be badly tested. Emotionally disturbed children who are not capable of dealing with the test situation may also be misdiagnosed. Some children may have developed inadequate cognitive skills because of severely disrupted early environmental experiences—those under institutional care, for instance. Such inadequacy may also exist in individuals from "disadvantaged" homes who exhibit a below-average IQ not only because of culture-biased tests, but also because they have suffered real and probably irreversible damage to their intellectual development from a profound lack of early stimulation.

Because of these diverse reasons for potential misdiagnosis, those working in the mental retardation field have in recent years increasingly looked to social and behavioral evidence of retardation in addition to test results. Among the behavioral differences that may be noted in the retarded, several relate to the tendency of retarded persons to react to immediate "here-and-now" stimuli, without proper regard for future consequences. They may respond to only one aspect of a situation; they may require more frequent "feedback" in terms of tangible results. A lessened capacity to anticipate future consequences may be evident; in some cases an individual may be able to verbalize such consequences, and yet be unable to put this awareness into practice. An example might be the inability to save money for the long term. There may also be evidence of inappropriate social behavior, because of differing emotional response, or a lessened ability to deal with complex social situations of which only a part is perceived. A retarded person may be more easily influenced by others, both because of a desire to please and weaker abstract and logical skills.

Obviously, many persons of normal intelligence have some of these problems. Thus behavioral differences in the retarded should be seen not as diverging discretely from "normal" behavior, and thus typical of the retarded alone. Rather, such differences must be judged on a continuous scale that takes into account human behavior in general. Many normal people do not adequately take into account future consequences; but in the retarded this tendency is likely to be more pronounced. Thus it is important to exercise great care in judging behavioral evidence as well as test evidence. Some behavioral indices, such as failure to develop linguistic skills at the appropriate ages, or serious difficulties in controlling the bladder far beyond the normal period, may *seem* obvious evidence. Yet there do exist cases of exceptionally bright children who have not talked until they were six years old, or who continued to wet themselves regularly even beyond that age.

Indeed, it must be emphasized that the fit between cognitive competence and behavioral adjustment is often problematic in the mildly retarded. To begin with, we must ask to what extent the various levels of cognitive development are associated with social adjustment. In exploring this question, let us return again to Piaget's framework. An important construct in that framework is *decentration*. This term means that children, as they develop, acquire the capacity to consider simultaneously more than one aspect of the situation—that is, to consider multiple perspectives of an event. In the arena of social interaction, this capacity is seen in the ability to take the "role" of another person in terms of the other's phenomenology (his precepts, concepts, motives, intentions, and needs). At the concrete operational level previously described, individuals become noticeably more adept at role taking. Preliminary evidence suggests that differential role taking bears an important relationship to interpersonal adjustment among the mildly retarded.[9]

Such evidence supports the idea that social competence

[9]For evidence concerning role taking among the mildly mentally retarded, see: G. G. Affleck, "Role-Taking Ability and Interpersonal Conflict Resolution among Retarded Young Adults," *American Journal of Mental Deficiency* 80 (1975): 233–236; G. G. Affleck, "Role-Taking Ability and the Interpersonal Competencies of Retarded Children," *American Journal of Mental Deficiency* 80 (1975): 312–316.

cannot be separated from cognitive competence, but many other factors are also involved in the social adjustment of persons with mild mental retardation, as is the case with persons whose IQs fall anywhere along the continuum. One must be cautious, however, about attributing social adjustment differences between retarded and nonretarded persons to the cognitive distinctions between them. Otherwise, we are led to the tautological conclusion that retarded persons behave the way they do *because* they are retarded.

Conversely, of course, if we focus solely on behavioral outcomes, and observe a similarity between levels of behavior of mildly retarded and nonretarded persons, we may miss the legitimate differences related to underlying intellectual competence. In many instances, the mildly retarded individual may be seen to be behaving as "intelligently" as a person of normal intelligence, but may have used a more primitive cognitive process to achieve behavioral adjustment. In this vein, Zigler has asserted that

> A clear distinction must be made between intelligence and the sheer manifestation of those adaptive or socially competent behaviors that are typically labelled intelligent. Behaviors indicative of social competence do not inevitably reflect normal intellectual functioning any more than the relative absence of such behaviors in the emotionally unstable, the criminal, or the social misfit inevitably reflects intellectual subnormality.

Thus, although behavioral evidence may assist us in trying to identify the retarded, it is no more an absolute criterion than intelligence tests. The mildly retarded may behave in a completely "normal" way in one situation, and yet be incapable of responding in an accepted manner in another. On the other hand, people of normal intelligence may well behave unacceptably in certain situations. It is imperative, therefore, that before labeling any given individual as retarded, as much evidence of as many different kinds as possible be marshaled. According to current practice, a judgment of retardation should not be made unless the presence of both low performance on standard intelligence tests *and* impairment of social behavior can be demonstrated. Even when both these indices appear to give clear evidence of retardation, many of us feel that caution needs to be exercised. Failure to exercise such caution can have extremely unfortunate consequences, even disastrous ones in situations where fundamental rights are affected—particularly, of course, when the question of sterilization is at issue. As we shall see, the court cases in this country involving sterilization of the retarded have too often been decided on the basis of a minimum of actual evidence.

In the course of this chapter we have talked more about the retarded child than the retarded adult. There are several reasons for this. First, in attempting to work toward a definition of retardation, it is important to make clear the presumed developmental differences between the normal child and the retarded child. In recent years a number of psychologists have begun to explore the continuing developmental psychology of the adult on the thesis that there are adult stages through which each of us must pass if we are to reach our full potential. Eventually, it is to be hoped that some of this work can be related to the life experiences and potential growth of the retarded adult. But at present, the vast majority of studies concerning the psychology of the retarded focus upon the childhood years. It is in the school setting that mild retardation is most often identified; it is in the school setting that intelligence and aptitude tests are first administered.

There are problems that arise from focusing on the childhood development of the mildly retarded. One of these derives from a central IQ-test construct—that of the *mental age*. A person's IQ is calculated as follows: mental age divided by chronological age multiplied by 100 equals IQ. Zigler has argued that, for example, the familially retarded person with a chronological age of 10, an IQ of 70, and a mental age of 7 ought to be viewed as being roughly at the same level of cognitive development as a child with a chronological age of 7 and an IQ of 100. But it is extremely important to recognize that this does *not* mean that the 10-year-old person with mental retardation behaves like a 7-year-old. Rather, this proposition refers to similarities in the cognitive structure of both individuals. Yet it is commonplace, among the general public, to refer to the retarded as "childlike," although the individual in question may be in his forties. It should be emphasized, therefore, that there are many ways in which the retarded adult is very different from a child. Many retarded adults develop social competencies that we would not expect of a child with the same mental age, and at the same time may not be able to make change of a dollar with the ease that we would expect of a child of 10; yet the same adult may hold a job as a gardener or handyman, working competently for 40 hours a week at tasks involving the use of machinery or tools that we would not entrust to a child. If the retarded were simply childlike, then the grave difficulties we encounter in attempting to ascertain whether or not a retarded adult is competent to vote, handle his or her own finances, marry, and bear or rear children would be obviated.

Finally, it should by now be eminently clear why this chapter is titled "Toward a Definition of Mental Retardation." "Toward" is the operative word in this context. If such a definition could in fact be laid down, many of our difficulties in determining what the rights of the mildly retarded should be would not exist.[10] We hope, however, this discussion will help to illuminate the reasons why we cannot arrive at easy or consensual answers when we attempt to strike a balance between the capabilities of the retarded and their rights in society. The difficulties in defining mental retardation have implications as well for attempts to educate mentally retarded persons. Yet the relationship between the adequacy of a definition of retardation and the appropriateness of various educational approaches is far from simple. The next chapter explores a range of ethical and social issues concerning the education of the mentally retarded, beginning with a brief historical account.

[10]For a more detailed exploration of the behavioral differences between the retarded and normal populations, see Chapter 9.

CHAPTER 3

Educating the Retarded

In 1798, a young man who had apparently grown to physical maturity in the wild, without human companionship, suddenly appeared in a French town. Jean Jacques Rousseau's concept of the "noble savage" was popular at the time, and the young man caused great interest. Adjudged retarded, he was given the name Victor and at first placed under the care of the physician, Phillipe Pinel, who specialized in mental disorders. Pinel, however, held the view that "idiocy" was incurable, and the French government subsequently allowed Jean Marc Itard to try to educate Victor. This effort was the first documented attempt at the education of a mentally retarded individual. Itard, who was aware of John Locke's ideas concerning the intellect as a storehouse, went on to develop the first self-help activities for the retarded. He made skillful use of a system of rewards for performance—a form of positive reinforcement, as it would be called today. Although he had some success with Victor, the young man's lack of speech development hampered Itard's work with him. It is unfortunately impossible to judge whether, in today's terminology,

Victor would be called culturally deprived, emotionally disturbed, or just mentally retarded.

Subsequent figures in the early development of educational techniques for the retarded included Edouard Seguin, Johann Guggenbuhl, and Samuel Gridley Howe. Seguin noted that in normal children standing, walking, and the use of the hands occurred at an early age, whereas the retarded were either delayed in the development of such skills or did not attain them at all. He worked with the severely retarded, teaching them to stand by means of a psychological learning technique that was an early version of the "escape-avoidance learning" still in use today. If the retarded person would not put forth the effort to stand, for instance, he was allowed to fall off elevated platforms. Thus the only way the individual could avoid the fear of falling was to perform the task required of him. These tasks were carefully sequenced for maximal learning by means of so-called task analysis. Seguin's goal was to prepare the retarded for social usefulness, an objective widely shared by fellow followers of Claude de Saint-Simon, the French social philosopher. The "Saint-Simonists" demanded that philosophy rid itself of abstract speculation and begin to apply ethics, laws, and economics to the reformation of society, with an emphasis upon the eradication of class distinctions and free education for all. Although Seguin believed that all retarded persons could be trained as socialists, he insisted that they not become slaves of industry.

Another tack was taken by Guggenbuhl, who pledged himself as "God-chosen" to begin full-time residential treatment of the retarded. Employing a special diet of foods, minerals, and herbal teas, coupled with baths, gymnastics, and massage, he achieved some success in teaching farming, animal husbandry, and basket weaving. He was perhaps the first to demonstrate the possibility of a labor pool of retarded people. Unhappily, he was also the superintendent of the first institution for the retarded to be closed because of scandal and poor management.

The concept of residential training schools spread

throughout Europe. Such schools were opened in the Netherlands in 1842, in England in 1846 and 1847, and in Germany in 1847. In America, Samuel Howe together with Dorothea Dix persuaded the Massachusetts legislature to found a public residential facility for the retarded in 1848. Howe, extrapolating from his earlier work with the deaf, perceived all mankind to possess an innate goodness which he believed needed only to be awakened and released. Curiously, however, he stated that he "played down" the idea of improvement, reporting that his major accomplishment was to arrest "the process of deterioration."

Seguin, whose socialist views made it necessary for him to leave France, came to America. He was more optimistic concerning the educability of the retarded than was Howe, but both men campaigned for the spread of residential schools for the retarded. Seguin held that the maximum student population in such a school for the retarded should be 150, with one staff member for every 5 to 20 students, with great reliance placed upon an all-powerful superintendent. In 1876, the U. S. Centennial, Seguin became the first president of the organization now known as the American Association on Mental Deficiency.

That same year a group of scholars held the first international meeting on mental retardation in London. Both the American group headed by Seguin and the London group noted that many defectives could be improved by "boarding out." But it was felt that some, the less promising cases, needed more protection, and it was proposed that there be established, "here and there, scattered over the country, villages of simple cities of refuge, havens in which all could live contentedly, no longer misunderstood nor taxed beyond their mental capacity." Both Howe and Seguin warned against this kind of separation, since, in Seguin's words, it would put the retarded "out of the reach of concourse, out of the reach of scientific men and means." Nevertheless, institutions were removed from population centers.

Again contrary to Seguin's ideas, large institutions became the norm. They were more economical, and inmates could work and earn their keep in them—just as had been the case in St. Vincent's Hospital in the 1600s. Howe had begun teaching the retarded, with a class of 10 students, in 1848, but within 40 years 15 states had institutions averaging 300 inmates apiece. These institutions reflected the philosophy that the retarded should be protected from the world and the world from them. The size of institutions continued to grow, and it was not until 1963 that President Kennedy's Panel on Mental Retardation recommended that institutions hold no more than 500 inmates.

Because our focus in this book is upon the mildly retarded, we will not be discussing institutional care except peripherally. Yet the development of education for the retarded over the past century, which was in many cases tied in with institutional care, has a direct bearing on the kinds of education offered to the mildly retarded in public schools at present. The themes that are evident in the brief history of education for the retarded that has been presented here are still very much with us. The context has changed, but many of the fundamental questions raised by such pioneers as Howe and Seguin continue to be debated.

Perhaps the most crucial and hotly debated question involves the matter of separating the mildly retarded from normal children in the educational process. In the public schools today there are two divergent approaches to educating the mildly retarded. In some schools they are placed in special, separate classes, but in other cases they are "mainstreamed," placed in classes together with normal children. Both these educational approaches have their strong adherents, and the points raised by both sides carry over into many other areas involving both the rights of the retarded and society's responsibilities in dealing with the retarded.[1]

[1]It should be noted that mainstreaming of retarded children did not develop solely out of right-to-education lawsuits. The concept was first promulgated by Maynard Reynolds, Professor of Special Education, University of Minnesota, and published in the *Journal of Exceptional Children* (March 1962).

For many years it was believed that retarded children profit from specialized educational programming carried out in segregated classrooms. However, the research in this area is far from clear. In fact, the best controlled study designed to evaluate the relative efficacy of placing mildly retarded children in special classrooms rather than in a regular educational setting, published by Goldstein, Moss, and Jordan in 1965, found no consistent pattern of academic advantage through placement in a special, segregated classroom. This study was based on comparisons among children whose mean IQ was 85 and below. The population studied consisted of children who had been in the first grade in 1958, with the study being based upon four years of data. Children scoring up to 85 were accepted as being mildly retarded at that time, but the cutoff point between mild retardation and low-normal intelligence has since been lowered, with a score of 70 now commonly accepted as the dividing line. This means that a significant proportion of the children in the study would be classified as culturally disadvantaged today, rather than as retarded. Additionally, the educational technology available 20 years ago was not as sophisticated as that available today. Numerous studies have established that mildly retarded children can learn much more rapidly and achieve higher levels of proficiency when modern behavioral management methods are used. In other words, it would not be surprising if no differences were found between mainstreaming and special educational placement when inadequate teaching methods are used.

Many advocates of mainstreaming, although admitting a need for special classes in some areas, stress the importance of the retarded child being in the company of "normal" students as much as possible. It is not denied that some of the retarded children may find this situation uncomfortable at times, both academically and socially. But it is pointed out that unless the mildly retarded can learn to "take their knocks" in the school situation, they will be much less prepared to deal with society at large when they become adults. In this connection, those concerned with statistical studies of mental retardation have long been aware that the number of "known" mentally retarded persons in any community drops sharply among those who are older and out of school. This fact would appear to indicate that once a young adult has left school and secured employment in the community, he may cease to be labeled as "retarded," and instead be accepted at his place of employment and in the community as just another young citizen. Many who feel strongly about the importance of mainstreaming believe that the more the mildly retarded child is exposed to the "real" world in which he will have to function if he is to seek employment, the greater are the chances that he will be able to deal with its exigencies.

If a child receives an education that consists entirely of special classes, according to this point of view, he will have no chance to develop the resilience he will need to deal with nonretarded people as an adult. The retarded child may be more protected in a school environment in which he encounters only other retarded children, but may not such protection deprive him of the opportunity to develop ways of protecting *himself*?

From another point of view, it can be argued that the real point is not whether children profit more from mainstreamed or segregated education. Rather the more germane issue would seem to be the provision of adequately trained staff, backed by appropriate curricula and teaching methods. This approach emphasizes that the educational plan, whether in an integrated or segregated setting, must be individualized and provide necessary support services. When these goals are achieved, as is being demonstrated by statewide projects in Texas and Vermont, mildly retarded children appear to profit from both forms of educational programs.

The contention that retarded children *do* require specialized services, in either setting, raises an additional question, however, as we can see by examining the three major objections to making distinctions between mildly retarded and nonretarded children in the educational process. The first objection is that making such distinctions not only leads to segregation but also to stigmatization and the violation of rights to which all citizens should have access. It is also pointed out that there are data indicating that providing specialized classes does not benefit mildly retarded children and that they are in fact just as well off being mainstreamed in everyday learning and living activities. The third objection is that since all of us exhibit some degree of one or more of the deficits characteristic of mildly retarded persons, the practice of making distinctions between normal and retarded is discriminatory and fails to provide equal protection under the law.

The issue of distinguishing the retarded from the nonretarded individual is hardly a moot academic exercise. It has been established by a number of studies that the stigmatization that was practiced for many years in this country has had disastrous consequences.[2] In response to the brutalizing and dehumanizing results of past discriminatory practices, litigation has led to radically different interpretations of any distinctions that may properly be made between retarded and nonretarded persons. Burt, for example, in interpreting the ruling in a Pennsylvania case (*PARC* v. *State of Pennsylvania*), has argued that

> any state program that segregates mentally retarded citizens as such from others is highly suspect, and . . . the courts will require states to treat mentally retarded persons indistinguishably from others, except in ways that are both very limited and very clearly beneficial to the individual.[3]

---

[2]The consequences of stigmatization are documented in the following works: E. Goffman, *Asylums* (Chicago: Aldine, 1961); B. Blatt and F. Kaplan, *Christmas in Purgatory* (Boston: Allyn & Bacon, 1966); M. S. Sargen, "Labeling and Classification," in M. Kindred, J. Cohen, D. Penrod, and T. Shaffer, eds., *The Mentally Retarded Citizen and the Law* (New York: Free Press, 1976); P. M. Wald, "Basic Personal and Civil Rights," in M. Kindred, J. Cohen, D. Penrod, and T. Shaffer, eds., *The Mentally Retarded Citizen and the Law* (New York: Free Press, 1976).

[3]For the interpretation of the cited Pennsylvania ruling, see R. A. Burt, "Beyond the Right to Habilitation," in M. Kindred, J. Cohen, D. Penrod, and T. Shaffer, eds., *The Mentally Retarded Citizen and the Law* (New York: Free Press, 1976).

Aside from the assumption that there are no behavioral differences between the retarded and the nonretarded, there are two aspects to Burt's argument that have specific relevance to the matter of educational programs. First, there is the implication that "segregation" is a relatively simple concept which would make it possible to clearly identify state programs that are indeed segregated. Second, there is the suggestion that segregated programs will be unconstitutional and therefore *not provided* unless they are *clearly beneficial* to the individual.

In respect to these implications, it should be pointed out that virtually all special educational services in some respect "segregate" the recipients of those services from others. Even where there is clear educational benefit for a student to spend part of his school day in a special classroom or working with a tutor, situations in which unique educational programming can be provided, such special help would necessarily involve a degree of "segregation." Are we therefore to abandon special tutoring and special classes for the retarded altogether? Or can such limited segregation be justified as "clearly beneficial"?

The complexities involved in any consideration of the concept of segregation can be demonstrated by reference to F. Goodman's 1972 paper, "De Facto Segregation," in which he states:

> If separation from faceless white students in other schools and other neighborhoods on the impersonal grounds of residence is damaging to a negro child's self esteem, the daily experience of being isolated from white students in his own school on the highly personal and pejorative grounds of ability must be infinitely more so.

If this argument is applied to the mildly retarded, some would draw the conclusion that partial integration of the mildly retarded child might well be more demeaning than total segregation in a separate school or classroom.

Moreover, some studies have shown that even when there is no explicit segregation of retarded children in mainstreamed classrooms, retarded children apparently distinguish themselves from nonhandicapped peers to a greater degree than retarded children in segregated classrooms.[4] This observation is supported by a recent finding that 60 percent of mildly retarded adults feel that retarded children should be educated in special classes in school.[5]

These observations are not intended as an argument *against* the integration of services, but rather to emphasize that the results of integration are mixed. Whereas integrated classrooms may lead some of the mildly retarded to view themselves more favorably, there are also clear indications that in such a situation other mildly retarded children come to see themselves as less like their nonhandicapped peers rather than more like them. Proponents of mainstreaming will argue that at the very least it places mildly retarded children in a situation that reflects the reality of what they will have to expect in later life. The job of the school, in this view, is to help mildly retarded children to move away from negative interpretations and qain more self-confidence, thus helping them to cope with reality. Those who stress the importance of at least some special programs in segregated classes will insist in return that the mildly retarded child gains more self-confidence in the company of other retarded children. Thus in exploring the consequences of either segregated or integrated programs, it is not a simple matter to determine whether or not given services are indeed beneficial.

Indeed, this matter has been a constant point of contention throughout our discussions. If we, working intensely within the familiar confines of a small group, could not reach accord on this point, it is obvious that other professionals

[4]For evidence concerning the degree to which retarded children distinguish themselves from their nonhandicapped peers, see W. J. Cagelka and J. L. Tyler, "Efficacy of Special Class Placement," *Training School Bulletin* 67 (1970): 33–68.

[5]In reference to the views of retarded adults as to the use of special classes, see J. Gan, A. T. Tymchuck, and A. Nishihara, "Mildly Retarded Adults: Their Attitudes toward Retardation," *Mental Retardation*, 15 (1977): 5–9.

working independently on different experimental projects are bound to come to varying conclusions reflecting a similar disparity of opinion. Whereas some of us believe that more rapid learning takes place in integrated classes, others feel that the reverse is true. Studies can be cited to support both arguments. Similarly, whereas some of us are particularly concerned that segregated classes are a form of discrimination, others of us are more disturbed by the possible stigmatization and exploitation that may occur when the retarded child is mainstreamed with nonretarded children. Which is the graver form of stigmatization: that which comes from being placed in a segregated class, or that which may be experienced as a result of comparing oneself on an everyday basis to nonretarded children—some of whom may intentionally or unintentionally make explicit their sense that the retarded classmate is encountering academic or other difficulties?

To complicate matters further, recent research on infants with known physical symptoms indicating retardation—Down's syndrome—has shown that they appear to profit intellectually from stimulation programs implemented very early in life, far before any meaningful assessment of later intellectual functioning can be made.[6] To conclude that it would be stigmatizing to provide such children with segregated infant-stimulation programs would also be to deprive them of later language and intellectual advantages derived from such programs. Even in the case of so-called cultural retardation, it appears that the gains made in early-intervention educational programs such as Head Start are lost unless special education services are provided on a continuing basis beyond the first three years of the program. In short, programs that are clearly beneficial may also involve a degree of segregation. To push for across-the-board elimination of such

[6]For evidence concerning early-stimulation programs for infants with Down's syndrome, see J. M. Horrobin and J. E. Rynders, *To Give an Edge* (Minneapolis: Colwell Press, 1972).

segregation could result in depriving the retarded persons, whose rights antisegregationists are trying to protect, of badly needed services.[7]

[7]Travis Thompson and Daniel Wikler conduct a fuller examination of the arguments regarding mainstreaming versus segregating of the mildly mentally retarded in Chapters 9 and 10, respectively.

CHAPTER 4

The Competence of the Mildly Retarded

Freedom of choice, or self-determination, for rational adults is a value that lies at the center of our moral tradition. This value, however, only began to occupy center stage in the Western world during the early seventeenth century. The Greeks did not have anything like our notion of the importance of the individual; their moral and political theories focused on the community and on a balance of interests and institutions within the larger society. Although the Greeks did have a well-developed theory of *virtue,* which applied at the individual level, they did not emphasize the concept of *rights* as we commonly use it to apply to individual needs, wants, or deserts.[1] But the rise of the ideology of individualism brought along with it the notion of rights—beginning with property rights—and also the concept of individual liberty.

The idea of individual freedom is sometimes referred to as "autonomy," but autonomy is a term that can engender confusion, since it is taken to mean a number of different things. For our purposes, let us therefore define autonomy as being roughly synoymous with self-determination or freedom from outside coercion or interference in matters pertaining to one's own life choices. The autonomy which most of us take for granted, however, is in a number of areas denied to the retarded.

We have noted that in many states the mildly retarded must submit to the guidance of others in making such key life decisions as living alone, entering into financial contracts, marrying, and having children. The standard reasons for denying full autonomy to the mildly retarded in making such decisions involve alleged dangers to the self or to others that might arise if the retarded were not restricted. These are not undisputed grounds, however. The danger to others is now often recognized as dubious, and the danger to the self is felt by some experts to be exaggerated. It might even be argued that the danger to the self is less than that posed by a paternalistic bureaucracy, endowed with broad powers but sometimes possessed of questionable wisdom and inconsistent motivation. Nevertheless, it seems likely that at least some mildly retarded persons would in fact do damage to their own interests if given full civil liberties, but can be protected from this harm by the restrictions mentioned above.

In the liberal tradition, the expectation of harm to the self is certainly a part of any strong argument for a paternalistic denial of liberties—to deny them merely to impose a benefit would be harder to defend. But to concede the existence of those who might do harm to themselves does not solve the dilemma. For persons of normal intelligence may also pose a danger or risk to their own interests. They can make impulsive contracts, enter into disastrous marriages, and choose occupations in which they are certain to perform poorly. Despite these possibilities, those of normal intelligence insist upon freedom of choice in such matters—not only the freedom to make good choices but also the freedom to make bad ones. The freedom to succeed also entails the freedom to fail. Although it is not absolute, a standard liberal principle allows us to do as we please as long as others' interests are not unfairly threatened. The fact that we may be on the verge of acting against our own interests is not generally sufficient excuse to restrict us.

Thus, the fact that some retarded persons pose a threat to their own welfare is not *in itself* a good enough reason to deny them the liberty to do so. The denial of liberty derives, instead, from an exception to the standard liberal principle. According to this line of reasoning, what makes it right to restrict a retarded person—and wrong to restrict a normal person posing exactly the same threat to his own interests—would seem to be the mental disability of the retarded individual. However self-destructive the nonretarded individual may be, it is claimed that he or she is capable of making decisions alone—of understanding what is at stake, weighing the alternatives, and taking responsibility for what happens as a result of the decision, even if the decision is as momentous as that of bearing and rearing a child. The mildly retarded, on the other hand, are held incapable of such understanding and deliberation by dint of their retardation. And thus decisions must be made for them, especially in psychologically and socially significant areas such as sterilization, just as they would be for the temporarily insane, the comatose, or others unable to reason.

But this argument is vulnerable to criticism at several points. One criticism, of course, involves the vagueness of the concept of "retardation." As we have seen in previous chapters, strong arguments can be made that the fact of a person having been labeled "retarded" through our social sorting mechanisms is by no means a sure guide to his intellectual abilities. Beyond this unsettled question, however, it is important to examine the presupposition that there are only two possible mental statuses: one of impaired intellect and one of unimpaired intellect, with the latter having a right to self-direction that is denied the former. For even if an intellectual deficit is recognized in the mildly retarded relative to the nonretarded, there is no obvious and compelling reason to attach such moral and legal significance to it. The moderately or severely retarded have such a deficit relative to the mildly retarded. And, more important, those of normal intelligence may have a deficit relative to the gifted.

Once it is recognized that there are in fact a host of cognitive statuses, further questions arise. Does there, for instance, exist a similarly large number of moral statuses corresponding to the various intellectual statuses? If average persons—now deemed normal—are "impaired" from the point of view of those of higher intellectual status, are they for this reason also subject to a paternalistic denial of civil liberties?

It would seem that if the intellectual superiority of those with normal intelligence legitimates our controlling the decisions of the mildly retarded, then the same difference in intellect would justify those of normal intelligence being regulated by the gifted. If we are to make decisions for the 3 percent of the population whose IQs fall below 70, why should we not have our decisions made for us by the 3 percent of the population whose IQs are above 130? Yet our putative right to self-direction is supposed to hold even when our decisions are poor and when others happen to know better. We are in the position, then, of using our relative intellectual superiority as our rationale for regulating the retarded, even though we reject the possibility of this same rationale being used upon us. Unless this apparent inconsistency can be resolved, it would seem necessary to either find new foundations for a paternalistic policy toward the mentally handicapped, or to abandon that policy.

The apparent inconsistency may be seen as growing out of a concept of mental capacity which may be termed *relativistic*. In the relativistic view, mental capacity is an attribute admitting of "more" or "less." The mentally retarded have less capacity than the average individual; the average person is in turn less endowed than gifted persons might be. No categorization of a group as "mentally impaired" will make sense, according to this view, unless it is understood as relative to the perspective of some other level. Those of average intellectual powers will thus be seen as impaired relative to the gifted, and the mildly retarded will be seen as well endowed relative to the severaly retarded. Intelligence thus becomes open-ended, like, for instance, wealth. Just as there is no point at which one becomes "fully wealthy"—only wealthier and still wealthier—so no one can become "fully intelligent." We may be able to distinguish various levels of mental ability through tests and the like. But no line drawn between mentally "impaired" and mentally "unimpaired" will, in the relativistic view, be anything but ad hoc. The line could be drawn somewhere else on the scale with equal justification.

The crux of the relativist view can be illustrated by reference to the specific components of what are believed to constitute the retarded person's deficit. The mildly retarded person, according to some authorities, is unable to think about or deal with more than one or two aspects of a complex situation. He or she is unable to defer gratification so as to make choices most likely to be of benefit over the longest run, or to foresee long-term consequences of present acts. He or she will be markedly less adept than those of normal intelligence in handling abstract concepts, as well as in making the kinds of judgments conducive to smooth social functioning.

The person of normal intelligence does somewhat better at all of these tasks. But it is plain that normal performance could be bettered. An exceptionally gifted individual, for instance, may have the ability to consider all the aspects of a very complex situation, to defer gratification as needed, to look far into the future, and to be at home with the loftiest of abstractions. In this context, "normal" will thus mean no more than "average," and "unimpaired" simply means as good as most others.

Any definition of normality in mental capacity which is based upon IQ scores will admit of a relativist interpretation. So does this statement of the American Association of Mental Deficiency:

> A person's mental capacity is determined by reference to whether he has the ability to manage his affairs with ordinary or reasonable prudence, is of sound mind, has demonstrated

> rational understanding or intellectual comprehension, is capable of making a full deliberation of matters presented to him, has the mental capacity to make choices and to formulate requisite judgments about those choices, has demonstrated an ability to engage in a meaningful intellectual process, has sufficient intellectual capacity to understand and appreciate the nature and consequences of a specified matter or to give intelligent consent to a specified procedure.

Clearly, these criteria could not be met even by very bright men and women if we set high standards for "full deliberation." Why, for that matter, should "ordinary or reasonable prudence" be enough? What is it about this "ordinary" prudence that earns those of average intelligence the right to be exempt from restrictions imposed by their superiors in intelligence, and yet allows those of average intelligence to restrict the rights of those less intelligent than themselves? From the relativistic point of view, of course, the answer would be that no such intrinsic right exists. Average mental capacity, which those of normal intelligence conveniently label "full' capacity, is simply what happens to be typical for our species at this moment in history. Obviously, the gifted would not be convinced that average intelligence was "unimpaired" or "full." As a consequence, the liberal principle previously cited—that a person of unimpaired intellect must be free to place his welfare at risk if he so chooses—loses its apparent reasonability.

The inconsistency could, of course, be resolved by abandoning the liberal principle. We could accept the rule that superiors may impose their paternalistic guidance upon those inferior to them—whether these be mildly retarded, normal, or even very bright persons. The relativistic view, however, can itself be questioned.

In countering the relativistic view, another approach may be taken. Full mental capacity can be seen as a "range property," to use the term elucidated by John Rawls in *A Theory of Justice*. A range property is one that is possessed equally by all who have it. But such a concept requires that a nonarbitrary threshold be determined, one such that all standing above it are equally endowed and all falling below are unendowed. The point of the relativist argument is that there can be no such line drawn when the property in question is general intelligence. Rather than disputing this claim, it may be more fruitful to seek a different, although related, property. The idea involved is simple and familiar, and will already have occurred to the reader. Mental capacity can be seen as a matter of *competence* rather than intellect, with competence being defined as the intellect's power in meeting a challenge. A given challenge may be wholly and fully met by the use of only a certain amount of intelligence, so long as the challenge is not too great. Although a person may have more intelligence than another, he or she may be no more competent at performing a great many tasks. His or her added intelligence is simply an unused surplus. Those lacking sufficient intelligence to perform a given task will be incompetent to perform it; whereas those having sufficient intelligence will be equally competent however great the difference in their intellectual levels.

This approach allows the determination of a nonrelative kind of mental impairment—at least in respect to tasks for which superior intelligence is of no additional advantage. Although added intelligence may increase the benefit to be derived from a given task or opportunity, a lesser talent is all that is needed to understand how to avoid harm. Geniuses may be no more adept than those of normal intelligence in determining the *safest* investments in the stock market—for instance, the preferred stock of the major corporations. On the other hand, the genius may be in a much better position to get rich because of his grasp of the potential of riskier investments. The threshold here lies between those able to comprehend and avoid the "downside" risks and those unable to do so. All those who can avoid such risks are equal in this respect. Relativism applies, in such a case, only to the capacity for realizing "upside" gains.

This conception of mental impairment would seem to support some use of the liberal principle. In the case of challenges for which a given level of intelligence is wholly sufficient, persons of superior intellect are not of superior competence. Thus, they could not use the principle's exception—which relates to impairment—to justify any abrogation of the decision-making power of those of average intelligence. The same will hold even for the second sort of challenge mentioned above, in which added intellect assists one only in realizing gain. As has been previously pointed out, the strongest argument for paternalism applies when the aim is to protect from harm, and not when it is to ensure a benefit. If a given level of intelligence is sufficient to avoid danger in a given task, those of greater intellect cannot use the liberal principle to restrict a person's liberty in hopes of increasing his gain.

If this argument is accepted, it allows the possibility of establishing a threshold, relative to certain sorts of tasks, that can be used to divide the mentally impaired from those of full capacity and competence. What is now needed, if this concept is to justify restricting the civil liberties of the retarded, is to show that this threshold happens to fall precisely at the level of intelligence just below what is termed "normal." The relativist claims to find no reason to suppose that the level of intelligence currently typical of our population is *particularly* conducive to the mastery of the key tasks a person faces in our society. Without the assurance that the average intelligence is indeed calibrated to the carrying out of such tasks in a way that the intelligence of the retarded is not, then it will continue to seem arbitrary to pick the average mental capacity as the one which confers a general right to self-direction regardless of outcome.

One reply to this question seems natural enough, but is nonetheless mistaken. The reply is that natural selection has rendered our capacities well suited to our tasks. It would be pointless for the relativist to inquire why our rate of respiration has just the right range and variation to serve us in our typical pursuits, or why our bodies perspire in response to overheating, thus maintaining a constant temperature within the normal range. The answer in both cases, of course, is that neither of these capacities is an accident. These traits, in addition to many others, are remarkable adaptations to our environment and the challenges it poses. In these, as in other physical characteristics, there is a threshold below which the organism is unable to thrive, and above which additional increments do not aid in avoiding destruction or deterioration. It is reasonable to assume that the same processes that contribute to the average human having the right physical capacities for survival also shape the endowment underlying the intellect.

Yet, however successful it may be in explaining why we have the respiratory rates or temperature-control mechanisms that we do, natural selection does not resolve our problems with mental competence. The challenges facing the intellect in modern society, in both complexity and difficulty, largely reflect the features of that society itself. The inheritable portions of human intelligence were no doubt fixed, however roughly, before the challenges that now typically confront us had developed. Evolution may well have supplied us with the mental ability to design and build shelter, or to distinguish edible foods from poisonous ones, but it cannot have been supple enough to ensure that we have the mental capacity to operate a spaceship or to pass the written examination for a driver's license.

These considerations do suggest what appears to be the correct reply, however. The reasons that the threshold of competence in our society falls at or just below the average are, first, that society itself has determined the level of difficulty required to perform key life tasks; and second, that it is beneficial to society for this level to be set just so as to render the average person competent.

The social component of a task like that of passing a driver's examination is obvious. It would be foolish to marvel at the wonders of nature for making us smart enough to learn the rules of the road. Those who devised the rules, and the examination to test a driver's knowledge of them, were responsible for gearing their difficulty to the capacity humans have developed as a result of evolution and environment.

What is more, this social component figures prominently in most decisions that have been denied to the mildly mentally retarded under laws restricting their civil liberties. For example, a person who enters a formal financial arrangement assumes an obligation to live up to the terms of the agreement and forswears the use of certain kinds of excuses. If a student takes out a loan, he obligates himself to repay the debt within a specified period of time and cannot bow out because of inconvenience, the fact that he could only secure a relatively low-paying job, or because he did not get such a good education with that loan. At the same time, certain excusing conditions may obtain: the safeguards embodied in bankruptcy laws can be seen as part of this complex transaction. These characteristics of financial agreements are socially defined, and are set at the level of intelligence necessary for understanding and taking responsibility for the risk. Insufficient intellect will prevent a person from anticipating the difficulties involved and thus incur the risk of going in over his head.

Essentially conventional, these arrangements might have been different. Society might have instituted rules allowing persons to annul contracts if they proved inconvenient or if the contractor misjudged his resources at the time of bargaining. Similar differences might have occurred in other areas—parents might have had to face no expectations of being charged with the care of offspring. Indeed, in some societies, both primitive and contemporary, communal child care sometimes removes much of the child-rearing responsibility from the blood parents. Under such conditions, persons whose mental powers were much weaker than the average would be competent to enter contracts, marry, and make other key decisions without regularly risking serious reverses which they could not predict or understand. The threshold dividing competence from mental impairment could thus be set much lower. Alternatively, of course, it could be set much higher. A society organized in terms of the very gifted would perhaps contain few of the safeguards for fallibility which our society has. Institutions would, accordingly, be even more valuable to those competent to partake of them, and as a consequence it would be necessary to restrict the rights of the person of average intelligence.

If, then, it is in theory within society's power to arrange itself so as to render the mildly retarded fully competent, why does this not occur?[1] Mere prejudice or selfishness—a society made up mostly of average persons concerned only for themselves—need not be the answer. There is considerable social utility, at least for those of normal intellect, in setting the threshold about where it is. Contracts which could be voided when misunderstood or inconvenient would not facilitate the exchange of goods. An appliance seller hands over the product in exchange for a piece of paper because he believes that payments will follow. If such expectation were lacking, no one, regardless of competence, would have a way of obtaining appliances without cash. The value of contracts and other arrangements—the very ones subject to control in our paternalistic restriction of the retarded—depends on their having features which make them hazardous to those with limited ability. Those of normal intelligence make the world safe for normality, but not necessarily safe for retardation.

The same holds true with respect to other abilities and capacities. The strength a person must have to be "unimpaired" is not set by biology but by the demands of society. It is, then, no surprise that those who design manual-gearshift mechanisms or set the size of grocery bags turn out products that presuppose something like the average amount of strength. Society benefits by setting the requirements this high. We could make do with levers and containers which even the very weak could handle; but these would undoubtedly be of less use to us. It is also worth nothing that as

[1]It should be noted that larger numbers of those who were once considered retarded are no longer considered so, because of the lowering of the cutoff point between low-normal intelligence and mild retardation to 70 on the IQ scale. Thus, to a degree, society has seen fit to render some "retarded" persons competent. Additionally, new educational and training techniques seek to render even those below the cutoff point competent.

current practice sets a threshold for physical competence, it renders all at or above that level equal in this respect. Those of normal strength are just as competent as the very strong in moving gearshift levers. The advantages of exceptional strength lie in other, more esoteric, pursuits. Yet, even if it is admitted that society adjusts the tasks required of individuals to a particular level that corresponds with average capacity, two problems remain in terms of judging an individual's competence. The first of these difficulties is that although an individual may be incompetent in some areas, that same person may be competent in others. The second difficulty, which we will come to shortly, is a moral one.

From a legal standpoint, competence is judged according to the individual's ability to acquire knowledge, to select and express his choices, and to make a rational decision—abilities which essentially involve the processes outlined in the previously quoted excerpt from the American Association of Mental Deficiency's handbook on consent. But although the legal concept is predicated on such psychological considerations as the acquisition of knowledge and the ability to make rational choices, there are no simple quantitative indices whereby psychologists can translate findings from psychological evaluations directly into legal constructs. Rather, inferences are made, whereby a professional judgment is made, on the basis of psychological data, regarding the degree of competence. The words "professional judgment" must be emphasized here. For in the course of this study, we have discovered—if we did not already know—that concerned professionals can come to quite different conclusions on the basis of the same information.

In extreme cases, it may be possible to conclude that an individual is wholly incompetent—as in profound mental retardation or acute psychotic conditions. But we are dealing here with mild retardation, which constitutes a borderline situation. And just as courts in different states have come to contradictory conclusions in sterilization cases, so the judgments of two different professionals testifying before the same court may be opposed or contradictory. It seems necessary to conclude, therefore, that in general a psychological evaluation is unlikely to yield a global assessment of incompetence. The best that such an evaluation can achieve is to help in determining competence *relative to a specific situation*. Even persons of above-average intelligence and free from serious emotional disturbances may be incompetent to deal with certain situations because of inadequate knowledge, experience, or training. For example, a nonpilot is likely to be totally incompetent to make decisions and take action regarding relatively simple aeronautical procedures, such as landing an aircraft.

Thus, in attempting to determine competence, there are three factors that must be taken into account. First, it must be recognized that competence may vary according to the type of decision to be made. Second, a person's capacity to deal with certain situations may vary according to age or to transient conditions involving emotional or motivational variables. Third, it must be considered whether or not the individual is capable of being trained to deal with a situation in the future even though he or she is not competent to deal with it at present. This last consideration is of particular importance with respect to the mildly retarded, and will be dealt with at length in later chapters as we come to terms with the particular issue of sterilization, where the question often turns on the mildly retarded person's capacity to serve as an effective parent. Moreover, this third consideration can affect the first two: if a person is capable of learning to be competent in additional areas, or if transient conditions are undermining present competence, then the first two points of judgment cannot be considered as fixed.

The need to focus on competence in the particular situation is emphasized by the fact that questions of legal competence encompass a wide variety of situations, including the right to enter into a contract or raise a family or give consent to being institutionalized, to undergo a medical procedure other than sterilization, and of course the matter of sterilization itself. If it were possible to clearly define the crucial elements of competence to deal with specific types of situations, criteria could be established whereby individuals could be evaluated to determine whether they do or do not possess the minimum psychological prerequisites to deal with given situations. Such definitions, although theoretically possible, have not been formulated. Furthermore, the situation becomes even more difficult when the competence of *classes* of persons—such as the mildly retarded—rather than of particular individuals is to be determined. To draw up such a definition of competence in respect to a class of persons, it would be necessary to establish criteria for competence in a specific type of situation, to go on to identify relevant common characteristics among a class of persons, and then to conclude that because of these characteristics, the persons in the class cannot meet one or more of the stipulated criteria. The trouble with stipulated criteria, of course, is that they may be biased—as they historically have been in respect, for example, to blacks—and that the conclusions will therefore be prejudiced.

Leaving aside the question of biased criteria, however, we can see that other difficulties exist in attempting to reach conclusions regarding incompetence of classes of people in respect to specific types of situations. For example, it might be determined that entering into financial contracts requires basic language and mathematical skills, that profoundly retarded persons lack such skills, and that, therefore, profoundly retarded people are incompetent to enter into financial contracts. Yet such blanket determinations would be much easier to apply to incompetence than to competence. The establishment of incompetence would merely require the absence of at least one necessary component, whereas the establishment of competence might require evidence not only of basic skills but of a sufficient level of skills to enter into certain types of contracts. For instance, even people of high intelligence often require the expert advice of lawyers and agents when they enter into complex contracts involving percentages, delayed payments, subsidiary rights, and so on. This fact may seem to return us to the relativistic dilemma discussed earlier in this chapter. But the point being made here is not that the mildly retarded may be only relatively less competent than the average person; rather it is that in judging the competence of a mildly retarded person, the assessment should be made in respect to particular situations rather than across-the-board.

The presence of mild retardation does not automatically establish a level of general competence or incompetence. Nor are data available to allow the conclusion that specific types of situations are inherently so complex that *no* mildly retarded person has the capacity to comprehend the consequences of giving his or her consent. The fact that a person is mildly retarded does alert us, however, to the *possibility* of incompetence relative to specific situations. This is because mildly retarded people are more likely to be deficient in attributes which may be essential to understanding specific situations. Therefore, when mental retardation is suspected, special provisions should be established to assess competence. The assessment, however, should be designed to determine whether the given person has the basic capacity to *understand* the particular situation under consideration, rather than whether or not he or she is mentally retarded.

Certain types of intellectual ability which are typically deficient in mentally retarded persons may be especially important in understanding the situations most likely to raise the issue of competence. Among these types of ability may be included abstract thinking, judgment, problem solving, the retention of information, and the understanding of the future consequences of actions. To the extent that these abilities are defective, competence may be questioned. Psychological testing and other types of clinical evaluation may reveal these deficiencies, particularly if the evaluators are alerted to the need to assess these specific abilities. Thus, in assessing competence, evaluators need to be aware of the particular abilities considered necessary to a full understanding of the situation under consideration. To request a psychologist simply to "determine the competence" of an individual can be relatively meaningless unless the assessment is performed in respect to the abilities required in particular situations. Only grossly impaired persons are likely to be found incompetent by all evaluators, but the evaluation of less severely impaired persons is likely to reflect the individual bias of evaluators. Conversely, meaningful evaluations are much more probable if the specific situation is described to the evaluator, and if he or she is alerted to the types of intellectual ability most relevant to an understanding of the situation and the making of a sensible decision.

In addition to considering strictly intellectual abilities, it is important to evaluate the degree to which the individual's decision making is likely to be impaired by other factors. Although a person may possess the intellectual capacity to decide wisely, other variables may interfere with his effective use of this capacity. As a result, he may be incompetent to consent to a particular procedure, although theoretically possessing the capacity to do so. Psychotic conditions which greatly impair judgment or the perception of reality are obvious examples. But severe depression or anxiety may also seriously undermine the effective use of intellectual capacity. Many mildly retarded persons—though by no means all—display personality characteristics which interfere with the effective use of their intellectual capacity and/or which render them susceptible to coercion. For example, retarded persons are generally considered to be more suggestible and submissive than nonretarded people. Research has indicated that they tend to conform, to feel helpless, to respond to others rather than to their own inner frame of reference, and to look to others for control of their destiny. If evidence of susceptibility to undue influence is present, then the competence of the individual to enter freely into contractual arrangement, for instance, would have to be seriously questioned.

Another common characteristic of retarded people which may raise questions regarding their competence is their tendency to give undue importance to present circumstances and to discount future consequences. Studies have indicated that retarded persons tend to be less concerned with the future than nonretarded persons. Long-term consequences are particularly likely to receive little consideration. Thus, particular care should be taken when consent is required for procedures which are irreversible or which present long-term risks.

Because of the suggestibility of the retarded, and their tendency to be unduly influenced by present circumstances, it is easy to persuade oneself that they need to be treated in a paternalistic way. Paternalism derives from the idea of treating other persons in a "fatherly" manner. The paradigm of paternalistic action is, of course, in our treatment of infants and young children. We believe that it is our duty as parents to protect our young children from harm by placing constraints on their behavior. We believe it is fully justifiable to interfere with their actions, choices, and decisions in order to prevent them from destroying themselves. With children there is a presumption *against* their ability to make the right decisions, and so paternalism becomes justifiable in the interest of protecting them against self-destructive decisions and actions. Yet once those children become adults, there is a presumption *in favor* of their ability to make the "right" decision. Even where we may think that their decision is mistaken in some way, the value that we place upon autonomy and individual liberties prohibits interference.

The fact that mildly retarded adults are in some ways "childlike"—not having progressed to the same levels of cognitive ability as normal adults—encourages us to take a paternalistic attidude toward them. Yet the mildly retarded adult is not *literally* a child. Therefore, we must also take into consideration the value that we place on individual liberty. In seeking objective criteria for deciding questions of competence, we are inevitably pulled in two directions at once, toward our sense that the retarded need to be protected and toward our belief in the right to autonomy. Thus we must take care that we do not err in either of two opposite directions: on the one hand, being too paternalistic, and therefore unjustifiably coercive, or, on the other hand, being too permissive, and therefore opening the way to self-destructive or irresponsible actions on the part of the retarded.

If we view the retarded as potentially *competent*, our assessment as to whether a given individual is actually competent must not be unduly influenced by our belief in autonomy. If we view the retarded as potentially *incompetent*, our assessment as to the given individual's actual incompetence must not be unduly influenced by our paternalistic concerns.[2] With this tension between paternalism and permissiveness in mind, let us examine how determinations of competence have been arrived at in specific court cases concerning the sterilization of the retarded. As often occurs when moving from the abstract to the particular, however, we will discover that the introduction of a new element—in this case the laws of the various states—complicates the moral questions involved.

[2]See Chapter 10 for a more comprehensive analysis of the case for restricting the civil liberties of the mildly mentally retarded.

CHAPTER 5

Involuntary Sterilization and the Law

A Review of Court Cases in the United States

The first attempt to pass a law mandating involuntary sterilization in the United States came in 1897, in a bill introduced in the Michigan legislature that failed to pass. This bill and those that were to follow in other states were based on the concept of *eugenics*. This term, meaning "good birth," was apparently coined in the 1880s by Sir Francis Galton, a cousin of Charles Darwin. The notion of selective breeding is, of course, a very old one—Plato discusses it in *The Republic*. But this general philosophical idea took on new strength with the rise of social Darwinism at the end of the nineteenth century. Darwin's scientific evidence concerning the "survival of the fittest" gave a new respectability to the idea of selective breeding, as well as to the notion of weeding out the "unfit." The

English philosopher Herbert Spencer went so far as to cite social Darwinism in defense of sweatshops, child labor, and starvation, while at the same time decrying public education, health care, and other social services that interfered with the elimination of those he regarded as unfit.

In the United States, the concept of eugenics was given an additional boost by Richard Louis Dugdale's study of criminality in the Jukes family. Although Dugdale stressed environmental factors, many readers were ready to conclude that the social ills of crime, pauperism, and disease were inherited, and that they were closely associated with intemperance, sexual promiscuity, mental illness, and "idiocy," to use the term current at that time. This conclusion was arrived at in spite of the fact that in Dugdale's study only one case of "idiocy" was reported out of the 709 subjects he studied.

Eugenicists offered a variety of solutions to what they saw as the problem of inherited criminality and idiocy. Such solutions ranged from euthanasia to the prohibiting of marriage between mentally defective people. The segregation of defective people in institutions, which was becoming increasingly common, was another solution. The state of Connecticut passed a law proclaiming that "Every man who shall carnally know any female under the age of forty-five who is epileptic, imbecile, feeble-minded, or a pauper shall be imprisoned for not less than three years." The same sentence awaited consenting females.

Within the institutions, castration of the males was often employed as a means of "protecting" inmates from the "evils" of sexual promiscuity, and as a way of ensuring a lack of offspring. But castration was not the kind of application of eugenics that could easily be sold to legislators—quite aside from the fact that it often had fairly serious psychological side effects. As often occurs, however, a new kind of technology was developed that made it possible for the eugenics philosophy to be carried out in a more acceptable way. The surgical procedure of vasectomy was invented. A Dr. Sharpe began using vasectomies in about 1890 at an Indiana state reformatory, eventually employing his new procedure on 600 to 700 boys. Castration also continued to be used—indeed, cases of castration still occur occasionally today—but it was on the use of vasectomies that the eugenics bills introduced into state legislatures were predicated.

After the defeat of the first involuntary-sterilization bill in Michigan, there was a hiatus of a few years. Then, in 1904, another bill was introduced in Pennsylvania; it passed the legislature but was vetoed by the governor. In 1907, however, an Indiana statute passed the legislature, was signed by the governor, and became law. Within the next three years, similar statutes were enacted in Washington, California, and Connecticut. In 1922, an association for the advancement of eugenics among cattle changed its name and became a national organization promoting eugenics for human beings. During the 1920s the eugenics movement reached its peak, and by the end of the decade 28 states had passed involuntary-sterilization laws.

Many of these laws were appealed to the courts. Public sentiment seemed to be fairly strongly against them, and when they were reviewed by the courts, a number of them were declared unconstitutional on a variety of grounds. The most common finding by the courts was that they constituted cruel and unusual punishment; in other cases, the laws were found unconstitutional on the grounds that they violated due process or deprived persons subject to them of equal protection under the law. It should also be noted, however, that even while these laws were on the books, in many states they were seldom utilized.

But then, in 1927, came a Supreme Court decision whose impact continues to reverberate to the present day. In the *Buck* v. *Bell* case, Justice Holmes wrote the opinion upholding an involuntary-sterilization statute for genetic reasons.[1] The Buck case was apparently what might be called a "friendly" test case. The superintendent of Virginia's State Colony for

[1] See Appendix for text of this decision.

Epileptics and Feebleminded Persons wanted to get a ruling as to whether or not the Virginia involuntary-sterilization statute would pass constitutional muster. The person to be sterilized was Carrie Buck, who was 17 years old at the time the case began, said to be the daughter of a mentally retarded resident of the Virginia State Colony. Carrie herself had recently had an illegitimate daughter who was alleged to be retarded. The word "alleged" must be stressed here, for later investigators who have gone back over the case have discovered that these and other factual allegations on which the case was based appear to be erroneous, as we shall presently see.

The case was first heard by the local circuit court, and then appealed to the Supreme Court of Virginia and finally to the United States Supreme Court. The circuit court found that the sterilization was constitutional. The decision was challenged at the state-supreme-court level, and Carrie Buck had the benefit of counsel throughout the case. Her sterilization followed a hearing and the decisions of the three courts, and finally took place in January 1928, when she was 21 years old. Carrie's lawyer raised a due process argument, and also the issue of whether the sterilization did not constitute cruel and unusual punishment. The court said it was not done as a punishment, and that in fact sterilizing the woman allowed her to be released to the community—an argument that is often still heard today.

There was also an equal-protection argument brought by Carrie Buck's lawyer, on the ground that the Virginia sterilization statute applied only to the residents of the state facility. But this argument, too, was rejected both at the state-supreme-court level and by the Supreme Court of the United States. An earlier Supreme Court decision, *Jacobsen* v. *Massachusetts*, had found that it was legal to have an involuntary-vaccination statute that applied only to children in school, even though that statute affected only a particular class of people, and this decision was cited by Justice Holmes in his opinion upholding the Virginia sterilization statute.

Justice Holmes wrote:

> The attack is not upon the procedure but upon substantive law. It seems to be contended that in no circumstances could such an order be justified. It certainly is contended that the order cannot be justified upon existing grounds. The judgment finds the facts that have been recited and that Carrie Buck is the probable potential parent of socially inadequate offspring likewise afflicted, that she may be sexually sterilized without detriment to her general health and that her welfare and that of society will be promoted by her sterilization, and thereupon makes the order. In view of the general declaration of the Legislature and the specific findings of the Court, obviously we cannot say it is a matter of law that the grounds do not exist, and if they exist, they justify the result. We have seen more than once that the public welfare may call upon the best citizens for their lives. It would be strange if it could not call upon those who already sap the strength of the State to make lesser sacrifices, often not felt to be such by those concerned. In order to prevent our being swamped with incompetents, it is better for all the world if instead of waiting to execute degenerate offspring for crime or to let them starve for their imbecility, society can prevent those who are manifestly unfit from continuing their kind. The principle that sustains compulsory vaccination is broad enough to cover cutting the fallopian tubes [citing *Jacobsen*]; "three generations of imbeciles are enough."

Although this decision has remained for 50 years as the controlling law in this area, it has been criticized over and over again on numerous grounds. To begin with, the accuracy of the facts in the case has been questioned. According to sociologists who went back over the origins of the case, Carrie Buck's daughter had been labeled mentally retarded by a Red Cross nurse at the age of one month. It was discovered that the child had died of smallpox in the second grade but that *at that time* she was a brighter-than-average student who was doing perfectly well. In other words, there may not have been "three generations of imbeciles" at all. Indeed, there were some questions about Carrie Buck herself—people were labeled imbeciles in those days without any distinctions being made among mild, moderate, and severe retardation.

The decision has also been strongly criticized in terms of the validity of its scientific base. Implicit in the decision is an assumption that if the mentally retarded are sterilized, then mental retardation will eventually be eliminated. This assumption is, of course, quite untrue. The figures available from a number of studies indicate that 80 percent or more of the retarded are born to *normal* parents. In a very small number of situations involving certain limited, carefully defined syndromes, it can accurately be predicted that mental retardation will be inherited, as indicated by chromosomal structure. But it is clear that mental retardation will continue to exist whether or not the retarded are sterilized.

Holmes's analogies have also been questioned. He speaks of those who sacrifice their lives for the state in times of war, and claims that we should thus be able to extract the lesser sacrifice of sterilization from the retarded. Yet the enemy who kills our soldiers, it has been pointed out, is hardly comparable with the child that might become a burden upon the resources of the state. The situation is more unlike than like. Obviously, too, the vaccination analogy presents difficulties: involuntary sterilization goes far beyond involuntary inoculation in terms of the abridgment of fundamental rights.

Critics of the decision also argue that Holmes used a very low standard in trying to see whether or not there was a violation of due process; when such fundamental rights are at stake, it is argued, there should be a higher standard of judicial scrutiny. Neither Holmes himself or the Supreme Court of that period can be totally blamed for this situation, of course. There has been considerable evolution in the law since then, and it is perhaps in some ways unfair to call so strongly upon our hindsight. But in terms of modern analysis, the constitutional reasoning in the decision might not hold up today. There is a fairly strong element of the philosophy of eugenics in the decision. The eugenics movement was then at its height, but our attitudes have changed considerably since then, and the philosophical content of the decision also seems to be of a rather low level.

Nevertheless, the impact of the decision has been very great. There have been attempts to in effect reverse the Buck decision in other sterilization cases that have reached the Supreme Court. That this reversal has not happened is in part attributable to the fact that the emphases of the arguments have changed. Rather than supporting sterilization on the basis of a eugenics-oriented philosophy, with the hope of improving the race, the courts have turned to arguments based upon the burden placed upon society by the need to raise and care for the retarded.

A typical case with this new emphasis was decided by the Oregon Court of Appeals in 1972. In this case, *Cook* v. *The State of Oregon*, the court approved the sterilization of a 17-year-old girl. The approval was based not on hereditary grounds but rather on the presumed burden to the state that would occur if the girl were to have children. It was held that this girl would be likely to have children that were neglected or otherwise dependent on the state, and this likelihood was found to be adequate justification for sterilization under Oregon law. Although recognizing that there are no clearly defined, generally applicable criteria for good parenthood, the court felt certain enough that this woman would not be a good parent that it was proper to sterilize her. We will be examining this case in the context of other decisions in the next chapter. But for the moment, it is sufficient to point out that the bases of the decision reflect a general trend in such cases.

In some other cases, various courts have dodged the precedents of the Buck case, and found ways of disapproving sterilization. Chiefly, these decisions against sterilization relate to situations in which the particular state does not have a sterilization statute. Such statutes exist in about half the states, but in those where they do not, the possibilities of getting around the Buck case are much greater. For instance, there is the Ohio case, *Wade* v. *Bethesda Hospital*. A judge who had allowed many sterilizations approved one for a mentally retarded, 18-year-old girl. When the girl turned 21, she sued the judge. A federal court found that there was no involuntary-sterilization statute in Ohio, and that in the absence of such a statute, the probate court had no judicial authority to allow sterilization to take place. The case survived a motion to dismiss and was heading for a trial when a fairly substantial settlement was made, money damages being paid by the judge to the plaintiff.

In March 1977, the United States Court of Appeals for the Seventh Circuit handed down a decision involving a similar situation, as embodied in the case of *Sparkman* v. *McFarlin.*[2] In this case a woman who had been sterilized by court order when she was 15 years old brought a civil rights action against the medical practitioners who had performed the sterilization, and against the Indiana circuit judge who had ordered it. The girl's mother had originally sought the court order for the sterilization, stating in her affidavit that her daughter was "somewhat retarded," although the girl attended public schools and had been "passed along with other children in her age level." The mother also claimed that without her knowledge or consent, her daughter had begun dating and staying overnight with older youths and men, and that the mother could not maintain a continuous observation over her to "prevent unfortunate circumstances." The judge signed the order for sterilization. No guardian was appointed to represent the girl's interest and no hearing was held. Moreover, the girl was not informed of the true consequences of her surgery, but was told that the purpose of the hospital visit was to have her appendix removed.

In 1973 the girl married, and two years later she learned for the first time that she had been sterilized. The couple brought action, seeking damages, contending that the girl's constitutional rights had been violated, while the husband claimed loss of potential fatherhood. The circuit court held

[2]See *Sparkman* v. *McFarlin*, 552 F. 2d 172 (CA 7 1977). This case was appealed to the United States Supreme Court; see Appendix (p. 232) for excerpts from the text of the Supreme Court's decision.

that the action of the judge who had ordered the sterilization had no basis in either law or equity, and was therefore taken without jurisdiction. The sterilization statute in Indiana applies only to the inmates of institutions; the superintendent of the institution, if a lawfully licensed physician or surgeon, is authorized to perform or cause to be performed sterilization treatment. But this girl was not in an institution, and no section of the statute gave judges the right to make such decisions or sign such orders.

Moreover, the court argued, the defendants could derive no comfort from the common law of other states. In general, as we have seen, courts have refused to allow sterilizations in the absence of specific legislative statutes granting such authority. In a footnote, the circuit court's opinion pointed out that in some cases the facts which might have warranted sterilizations had been quite compelling, but still had been disallowed in the absence of specific statutes. For example, in *Franzier* v. *Levi*, the subject was an adjudged incompetent woman, 34 years old but with the mentality of a six-year-old. This woman was the ward of her parents, who were also supporting her two illegitimate children, both retarded. The parents claimed that they could not bear the economic burden of any more children. Even in these circumstances, however, the court had found that it could not authorize sterilization because of the lack of statutory mandate.

The court concluded:

> If we were to say that jurisdiction existed to order sterilization without adherence to the requirements of institutionalization and procedural due process mandated by the Indiana legislature, we would be sanctioning tyranny from the bench.

In addition, the opinion found the action of the judge who signed the sterilization order to be an illegitimate exercise of his common-law power because of his failure to comply with elementary principles of procedural due process. Here a juvenile was ordered sterilized without the taking of any steps to ensure that her rights were protected—not only was the plaintiff not given representation, she was not even told what was happening to her.

It should be noted that sterilization itself is not ruled out in this opinion, but only sterilization in these circumstances in which state law did not confer such authority. In a number of other cases the issue of a state's right to authorize sterilizations, as embodied in the Buck case, has been avoided through findings that a state statute was lacking in the necessary due process elements, such as the right to counsel and a hearing, the right to put in evidence of one's own, and to appeal if appropriate. Essentially, in such cases, the way was left open for legislatures to rewrite the laws to provide such protection.

A major case which involves a narrowing of circumstances in which sterilizations can be authorized but which leaves standing the right of legislatures to enact sterilization laws is *North Carolina Association for Retarded Children* v. *State of North Carolina.*[3] The North Carolina statute that was challenged in this case authorized both voluntary and involuntary sterilizations. It applied to mentally defective persons housed in state institutions *and* those who were not residents in state institutions. In respect to a resident who was confined in a state institution, the person in charge of the sterilization procedure was the director of the institution. For retarded persons not in state institutions, the key official was the county director of social services. Sections 35–39 make it the *duty* of the petitioner to institute sterilization proceedings under the following circumstances:

1. When he feels that sterilization is in the best interests of the mental, moral, or physical improvement of the retarded person.

2. When he feels that sterilization is in the best interests of the public at large.

3. When, in his opinion, the retarded person

> would be likely, unless sterilized, to procreate a child or children who would have a tendency to serious physical, mental or ner-

---

[3]See Appendix (p. 220) for text of this decision.

vous disease or deficiency; or, because of a physical, mental, or nervous disease or deficiency which is not likely to materially improve, the person would be unable to care for a child or children.

4. When the next of kin or legal guardian of the retarded person requests that he file the petition.

The court concluded that subparagraph 4 of Section 39 was irrational and irreconcilable with the first three paragraphs.

> The first three paragraphs make out a complete and sensible scheme: that the public servant concern himself *either* with the best interest of the retarded person *or* the best interest of the public, or both, *and* that he act to begin the procedure *only* when in his opinion the retarded person would either likely procreate a defective child or would himself be unable to care for his own child or children. All of this makes sense. The fourth subparagraph does not. Instead, it grants to the retarded person's next of kin or legal guardian the power of a tyrant: for any reason, or for no reason at all, he may *require* an otherwise responsible public servant to initiate the procedure. This he may do without reference to any standard and without regard to the public interest or the interest of the retarded person. We think such confidence in *all* next of kin and *all* legal guardians is misplaced . . . . We hold this subsection four unconstitutional as an arbitrary and capricious delegation of unbridled power and a correspondingly irrational withdrawal of responsibility sensibly placed upon the director of the institution or the county director of social services by the other three coherent and compatible subparagraphs.

Although this opinion found the statutory scheme constitutional with the execption of subparagraph four, its analysis of the questions concerning the right of the state to mandate involuntary sterilizations is perhaps as thorough as in any case that has yet arisen. For instance, there is a very clear statement in the opinion to the effect that most competent geneticists "now reject social Darwinism and doubt the premise implicit in Mr. Justice Holmes' incantation that . . . three generations of imbeciles is enough.' " But even though it dismisses this basis for mandating sterilization, the opinion makes some statements on the other side of the question as well, drawing a number of hard balances between the two sides.

"But however doubtful is the efficacy of sterilization to improve the quality of the human race," the opinion goes on,

> there is substantial medical opinion that it may be occasionally desirable and indicated . . . . We think it is a fair statement, from the expert testimony we have heard and read, to say that the best opinion presently is that rarely would a competent doctor recommend involuntary sterilization, but that he might do so in an extreme case. As a corollary to that proposition, it is also fair to say, we think, that prevalent medical opinion views with distaste even voluntary sterilization for the mentally retarded, and is inclined to sanction it only as a last resort and in relatively extreme cases. In short, the medical and genetical experts are no longer sold on sterilization to benefit either retarded patients or the future of the republic.

Furthermore, the opinion states that "some general propositions must be regarded as established by the evidence in this case. We emphasize that the following statements do not apply to all or even a majority of the plaintiff class." The opinion then lists a number of points that have considerable bearing on the problems we are focusing upon in this book. First, it notes that mental retardation sometimes has as its cause identifiable genetic defects, and that under some circumstances it is within the capability of modern medicine to establish that the genetic defect is inheritable, and that a significant probability exists that the offspring will inherit that defect.

Second, the opinion argues that mental retardation can in some cases be traced to an environment which blocks or shrinks the mental and intellectual development of the child; as a corollary, therefore, it is stated that in some cases it is possible to predict with substantial accuracy that a mentally retarded person would be incapable of discharging the responsibilities of parenthood because that person would be unable to create a nondetrimental environment.

Third, it is stated that although mentally retarded persons may be entitled to express themselves sexually, it can be determined in some cases that they do not understand or cannot appreciate the natural consequences of sexual activity, and would not realize that a child might be the result. Fourth, the point is made that some mentally retarded persons who are sexually active may not want children, and that although many sexually active retarded persons are capable of employing various methods of birth control, some are not. Finally, the opinion holds that in rare and unusual cases it can be medically determined that involuntary sterilization is in the best interests of either the mentally retarded person or the state, or both.

Thus this decision, although it narrows the circumstances under which voluntary sterilization may be carried out, by no means concludes that there cannot be an involuntary-sterilization statute. It to some extent shifts the rationale of the Buck case, saying that although some of the scientific underpinnings of that case were inaccurate, there still remain sufficient grounds for a more narrowly drawn statute to pass constitutional muster. This decision takes on added importance in that it seems representative of how far most courts are prepared to go in regard to the sterilization question at the present time. It typifies the tensions in the area and indicates that the fundamental moral questions involved in involuntary sterilization are still not being fully addressed by most courts.

There are three other cases that need to be examined in some detail. In two of these cases, the court's decision granted the authority for sterilization; in the third, the sterilization was prohibited. The importance of these cases lies in the fact that, taken together, they illustrate that the granting or denying of authority to sterilize is not necessarily based upon the particular capabilities (or lack of capabilities) of the retarded person in question.

The first of the cases decided in favor of sterilization has already been mentioned: *Nancy Rae Cook* v. *State of Oregon*, decided by the Oregon Court of Appeals in April 1972. The plaintiff in this case was a 17-year-old girl with a history of severe emotional disturbance. At age 13 she had been declared a ward of the court and was taken out of her home under circumstances indicating that she had been physically and sexually abused by her family for some time. In the intervening four years, she was placed in two foster homes, a juvenile detention home, a state hospital, and a special school. A petition was filed with the Board of Social Protection, requesting permission for sterilization, after the girl had engaged in a series of indiscriminate and impulsive sexual involvements while she was in the hospital.

Testifying in favor of the sterilization was a psychiatrist who specialized in child guidance, and who had followed the girl's case since she became a ward of the court. His uncontradicted testimony was that she would never be able to provide the parental guidance and judgment that a child requires, even though she might be able to master the skills necessary to take physical care of herself and a child. The psychiatrist based this conclusion on the girl's lack of emotional control, her consistent low scores in areas of judgment on psychological tests, and the likelihood that she would abuse a child. He testified further that both mental illness and mental retardation were contributing factors to her behavior, and were interrelated.

An Oregon statute allows for involuntary sterilization of individuals whose children will become neglected or dependent as a result of their parent's inability—by reason of mental illness or mental retardation—to provide adequate care. The court argued that the state's concern for the welfare of its citizenry extends to future generations, and that the state has sufficient interest to order sterilization when, as was found in this case, there is overwhelming evidence that a potential parent will be unable to provide a proper environment for a child because of mental illness or mental retardation. The court of appeals therefore affirmed the sterilization order of a circuit court.

But while the Oregon case was decided in terms of the welfare of the state, a New York case in 1976 resulted in the authorization of a sterilization on the basis of a very different rationale. *In the Matter of Frances Sallmaier* (N.Y., Queens County, Supreme Court), involved a 22-year-old woman whose mental retardation resulted from organic brain damage and was irreversible. She functioned at a six or seven-year-old age level and had many phobias, as well as a proclivity for encounters with males. Her mother applied for an order authorizing her to consent to a sterilization order on behalf of the daughter.

Since 1918, New York State has not had a statute authorizing the sterilization of individuals. The judge therefore held that the court's jurisdiction arose not by statute but from common-law jurisdiction to act as *parens patriae* with respect to incompetents. In his opinion, the judge cited the rationale used in an earlier case:

> the decision to exercise the power of *parens patriae* must reflect the welfare of society, as a whole, but mainly it must balance the individual's right to be free from interference against the individual's need to be treated, if treatment would in fact be in his best interest.

A court-appointed psychiatrist diagnosed the young woman as having severe mental retardation with marked infantile thinking, behavior, and attitudes, and stated that she was unable to understand abstract concepts and did not know the difference between a man and a woman. The psychiatrist was further of the opinion that pregnancy would have a substantial likelihood of causing a psychotic reaction. Great weight was given to the psychiatrist's opinion concerning the possibility of a psychotic reaction to pregnancy, and the court concluded that it would be in the best interest of the young woman to have a sterilization performed.

The young woman whose sterilization was authorized in New York had an IQ of 62. In Missouri, however, the sterilization of a young woman with an IQ of 50 was disallowed. The Missouri case, *In the Interest of M.K.R.* (Supreme Court of Missouri, 1974), was heard on appeal, following a judgment of the Juvenile Division of the Circuit Court of St. Louis County. The higher court reversed the decision of the juvenile court, which had originally authorized the sterilization of M.K.R. The child's mother had filed a petition claiming that the child was mentally retarded and unable to care for herself. The girl was a student at a learning center, and the personnel in charge of the center had recommended sterilization to avoid possible pregnancy. The mother said that she believed sterilization would be in the best interests of the child.

The evidence on which the trial judge of the circuit court had based his decision included the fact that M.K.R. had trisomy 22 (an extra chromosome, in the 22 series), an IQ of approximately 50, and severe learning, emotional, neuromuscular, and motor problems. It was stated that the girl had problems with her bladder and bowels and was unable to care for herself. She was said to be "overly friendly," with unpredictable behavior patterns, and thus faced with the constant threat of being assaulted and ravished. She was unable to care for herself during menstrual periods, and did not understand their significance. It was stated that should she become pregnant, there was a strong likelihood that her child would also be abnormal, and that because of her mental retardation she would be unable to care for a child. Based on these findings, the trial judge concluded that sterilization "would be conducive to the child's welfare and to the best interests of the state."

This decision was reversed by the Missouri Supreme Court on the ground that no section of the juvenile code conferred on the juvenile court the jurisdictional power to order or authorize the sterilization of a child. The opinion stated:

> We are faced with a request for sanction by the state of what no doubt is a routine operation which would irreversibly deny to a human being a fundamental right, the right to bear or beget a child. Jurisdiction of the Juvenile Court to exercise the awesome right of denying that right may not be inferred from the general language of the . . . code . . . . Such jurisdiction may

> be conferred only by specific statute. Whatever might be the merits of permanently depriving this child of this right, the Juvenile Court may not do so without statutory authority—authority which provides guidelines and adequate legal safeguards determined by the people's elected representatives to be necessary after full consideration of the constitutional rights of the individual and the general welfare of the people.

The cases we have outlined in this chapter have focused upon involuntary sterilization.[4] In a subsequent chapter we will be dealing with the matter of "voluntary" sterilization of the retarded, but first it is necessary to confront a host of questions raised by the members of our research group in respect to the involuntary-sterilization cases presented here.

[4]See Chapter 11 for a fuller discussion of the legal issues involved in the question of involuntary sterilization.

CHAPTER 6

Involuntary Sterilization and the Rights of the Mildly Retarded

In discussing the involuntary-sterilization court cases, some members of our group were particularly concerned with the discrepancies between decisions in different states, noting a lack of a consistent moral or philosophical point of view. The question of whether or not involuntary sterilization ought to be allowed under *any* circumstances was broached, revealing a number of differences of opinion among the group members as to the possible existence of circumstances in which the retarded might indeed "benefit" from sterilization. A particularly telling debate arose over the difficult matter of judging in advance the ability of a retarded person to function as an adequate parent.

To begin with, the point was made that an examination of the cases cited shows rather convincingly that an injustice is wrought by a legal system that must rely on different—and often contradictory—statutes in different states. Even this relatively small number of cases is sufficient to demonstrate the variation that currently exists in both legislation and judicial opinion in respect to involuntary sterilization. What is most striking is not simply the variation in the laws of the different states—since that is a feature of life in the United States mandated by our Constitution. But the differences from state to state result in the performance of seemingly unwarranted sterilizations in one place, whereas in another place sterilizations that appear much more clearly warranted are ruled out. Regardless of the rightness or wrongness, in principle, of laws that permit or require involuntary sterilization, a clear injustice becomes evident when a comparison is made between the Sallmaier case in New York and the Missouri case, *In the Interest of M.K. R.*.

In the New York case, the retarded young woman is described as having "severe mental retardation"—this being the diagnosis of the court-appointed psychiatrist. Yet the report of this case also notes that the young woman had an IQ of 62. This is hardly an IQ level that warrants the label "severe mental retardation;" rather, it would put the young woman at the "mild mental retardation" level.

The discrepancy between the measured IQ of 62 and the "severe" label suggests one of three things. First, it could suggest that the court-appointed psychiatrist had little knowledge or experience in the field of mental retardation. If this were true, then the psychiatrist should not have been appointed by the court to make a diagnosis. Even if the psychiatrist was aware that an IQ of 62 is indicative of mild retardation, his clinical evaluation that the young woman had "marked infantile thinking, behavior and judgment" should have been backed by additional evidence in order to show why he discounted the adjudged IQ level—although it is possible that the judge himself was at fault here for not including such evidence in his opinion. It is also possible that regardless of the significance of the young woman's IQ, the psychiatrist simply felt that it was appropriate to accede to the mother's wish that her daughter be sterilized, and so testified that the young woman was "severely retarded" to increase the likelihood that the judge would authorize the sterilization. The fact that the young woman was unable to understand abstract concepts may be supportive evidence of her retardation—but as several members of our research group have previously noted, a lack of understanding of abstract concepts does not necessarily indicate lack of competence in all areas. Finally, the statement that the young woman did not know the difference between a man and woman appears to be at odds with the claim that she had a proclivity for encounters with males; why should she be so sexually interested in males if she was not aware of sexual differentiations? This contradiction could indicate that the evidence was in a sense being stacked against the young woman, with statements being made without regard to consistency but rather with an eye to swaying the judge.

It seems likely that such contradictions and inconsistencies would have been challenged if the young woman had been represented by counsel. Both the lack of counsel and the absence of a sterilization statute in the state of New York would seem to provide grounds for appeal to a higher court. Such an appeal was not made, and so the authorization for sterilization stood. It cannot be said whether an appeal would have brought a reversal. But it can be noted that in Missouri the state supreme court *did* reverse the lower court authorization for the sterilization of M.K.R. It is ironic, however, that the evidence in the Missouri case offers a much stronger presentiment that sterilization might be warranted than was true in the New York case.

M.K.R. is said to have an IQ of approximately 50—which would put her at the moderate retardation level. It is stated that she is unable to care for herself in several important respects, having problems with her bladder and bowels, and unable to understand or deal with the exigencies of her menstrual periods. These facts alone strongly suggest that she is less capable of bearing and rearing a child than the young woman in the New York case. Yet here the sterilization was disallowed because of the juvenile court's lack of jurisdiction.

The different outcomes of these two cases—where it would appear that opposite resolutions would have been more appropriate—indicated to some of us that we cannot look to the courts for *moral* guidance in determining whether or not involuntary sterilizations violate the rights of the retarded. Law and morality *may* coincide, but they do not always do so. If law and morality did always coincide, then, in the light of these cases, what is morally right in New York is morally wrong in Mississippi. There is no problem with noting that what is *legal* in one state may be illegal in another. But that, precisely, is the difference between morality and legality. What is more, laws are often changed for what are believed to be moral reasons. For instance, we do not now believe that it was ethically justifiable to cut off the hands of thieves in past centuries, even though the laws of that time permitted such cruel and inhumane punishment of criminals. Even in our own time, laws are changed in ways that reflect a revised moral point of view. For example, in the North Carolina case, in which a portion of the existing law was found unconstitutional, the court's opinion concerning the fourth subparagraph is couched in moral language:

> It grants to the retarded person's next of kin or legal guardian the power of a tyrant; for any reason, or for no reason at all, he may *require* an otherwise responsible public servant to initiate the procedure. This he may do without reference to any standard, and without regard to the public interest or the interest of the retarded person. We think such confidence in all next of kin and all legal guardians is misplaced.

Since this section of the law was struck down on the basis of a moral argument, the implication is that the law, while it was in effect, was morally unsound. Yet it was the law, and presumably was felt to be morally sound by the legislators who framed it. What we have here, obviously, is a difference in moral perspective. In a pluralistic society this situation is only to be expected; but the fact that it must be expected does not mean that we cannot deplore those circumstances in which the result is injustice—as some of us believe occurred in these various sterilization cases.

There is a further difficulty in the fact that even when a strong moral argument is set forth, it may still in some cases result in a faulty decision. For instance, the Oregon statute concerning involuntary sterilization is predicated upon society's welfare. A good argument can be made that there are circumstances in which the welfare of society must be placed above the rights of the individual. In the Oregon case, the court determined that the welfare of society extended to future generations, and that a retarded individual who is clearly shown to be incapable of raising a child should be liable to sterilization. But even if one agrees with this line of moral reasoning, one may still find that the facts in the particular case at hand did *not* "clearly show" that the girl in question was incapable of raising a child. For some of us, this is the strongest reason possible for feeling that involuntary sterilization should be ruled out altogether—if it were, nationwide, then there would be less possibility of the kinds of injustice that become apparent when the various cases cited are compared. As matters stand, if it is to be claimed that law and morality *do* coincide, then sterilization is both morally right and morally wrong, depending upon the laws of the state in which the retarded person happens to live. To some of us, this contradiction seems insupportable.

Yet others among our group, in reviewing these cases, were prepared to argue that sterilization can indeed be morally right in some cases and morally wrong in others, depending upon particular circumstances. One of the chief arguments put forward to support this point of view is that in some cases involuntary sterilization fosters rather than denies the membership of the mildly retarded in the social community, and indeed in the moral community. Membership in the moral community means that a person is taken to be morally responsible for his or her actions in life, and is to be held responsible by the rest of the community for doing so.

The argument that involuntary sterilization fosters participation in the social and moral communities rests upon several observations. First, many mildly retarded people are capable of engaging in and taking pleasure in heterosexual intercourse. Second, for some mildly retarded people, sexual activity can be integrated with emotional aspects of affection, which can in turn contribute positively to personal and social fulfillment. Leaving aside for the moment questions of pregnancy, childbearing, and child rearing, an active heterosexual life can enrich the existence of the mildly retarded in much the same way as it can that of the average person. Other things being equal, mildly retarded people can benefit from and have a right to both sexual activity and the social forms, such as marriage, that sexual relationships can involve.

But pregnancy, childbearing, and child rearing are all elements that contribute to making matters unequal. For many mildly retarded women, the physiological and emotional changes that take place during pregnancy, and the strain of childbirth itself, are often experienced as disorienting and even terrifying traumata. To the extent that a retarded man participates in the process, he too can be disoriented. Moreover, child rearing is sometimes beyond the capacities of mildly retarded people. If there is not a reasonable expectation that children will receive minimal care, should not steps be taken to ensure that they are not conceived?

The prevention of conception by usual forms of contraception is often difficult for retarded individuals to manage—in some cases because they do not fully understand the significance of contraception, and in other cases because of the difficulty that many retarded people have in taking into account long-term consequences and in delaying gratification. All these factors may be combined, of course. Sterilization is the only form of contraception that is permanent, and which will free the retarded from all risk of pregnancy.

Advocates of this rationale for involuntary sterilization noted the need for several conditions or safeguards to protect the retarded from unwarranted sterilizations. First, it should be fully ascertained that those considered for involuntary sterilization indeed fall into the category of the mildly retarded. Although this may seem an obvious safeguard, it is important for two reasons. One reason is that there have been cases where individuals were sterilized without adequate proof that they were actually retarded. The *Sparkman* v. *McFarlin* case cited in the previous chapter, in which a young woman was sterilized without her knowledge at the age of 15, and later, after marrying, brought suit against the judge who had authorized the sterilization, is an example of this kind of situation. In this case, the only evidence introduced to establish the fact of the girl's retardation was her mother's statement to that effect. A second reason for including this safeguard, and for specifically insisting that the individual fall into the *mildly* retarded category, is to maintain the consistency of the argument. For, obviously, this argument cannot apply to those who are so severely retarded that they must remain institutionalized. To sterilize the severely retarded might be to the benefit of the institution itself; it might prevent the conception of unwanted children; and it might even be to the benefit of the retarded. But such sterilization would not rest on this argument; it would not make it possible for the profoundly retarded to be released to the community, nor leave them free to engage in sexual intercourse according to their own free will. Indeed, since most of the severely and profoundly retarded appear to have little or no sex drive, there are also substantive reasons for not applying this argument to their case. The argument is based upon the idea that sterilization would be of direct benefit to the individual, and thus must be applied only to the mildly retarded.

A second safeguard proposes that those to be sterilized be capable of engaging in and taking pleasure in heterosexual intercourse. Once again, this caveat is necessary to the consistency of the argument. A third condition calls for the establishment of evidence that in each particular case the retarded person is likely to suffer disorientation and possible trauma because of pregnancy. If this fact cannot be established, and there is good reason to think that the individual could cope with pregnancy and childbirth, then a fourth condition is brought into play. Here, it would be necessary to show that the individual's potential children could not be cared for competently and loved to maturity by the retarded person or in some alternate situation.

The rationale that sterilization would allow the retarded person to engage in sexual intercourse without fear of pregnancy and thus facilitate the retarded person's participation in the community at large can also be looked at from a philosophical point of view. In that tradition of Western ethical theory which takes the dignity of the human individual most seriously, one of the central concerns has been that of the moral community. Membership in the moral community means that a person is taken to be morally responsible for his or her actions, and is to be held responsible by the rest of the community for such behavior and life plans. The human dignity conferred by acceptance within this moral community is endangered whenever the individual comes to be treated as a thing rather than a responsible agent. This may happen when someone or some group treats a person merely as a means toward their own ends; which was, for example, Immanuel Kant's particular worry. But it may also happen—and often has happened in respect to the retarded—when the community simply fails to recognize the individual as a moral agent. In such situations, people's behavior is usually explained in such a way as to shift *responsibility* for that behavior away from the individuals themselves and onto other causes. In a strict philosophical sense—deriving from Aristotle—violence is done to people when they are prevented by external forces from fulfilling their basic or natural goals. One form of such violence is to prevent a person from exercising membership in the moral community.

Because of the incapacities associated with mental retardation, special care needs to be taken to ensure retarded persons as full a membership in the moral community as possible. Thus it is sometimes argued that to sterilize the retarded involuntarily is to do them unnecessary and dehumanizing violence. It is to regard them, first of all, as irresponsible in terms of deciding for themselves as to the desirability or need for sterilization, and so to exclude them from the moral community in this respect. Second, it is to assume that in the areas of sexual intercourse, childbearing, and child rearing their lives are so controlled by irresponsible forces that it is better for them to be managed like objects in these areas. Third, it is possible and even likely that sterilization may be sought for the retarded in order to make their custody easier; in such cases, the retarded come to be treated as means rather than ends in themselves.

These objections can perhaps be answered through a further exploration of the nature of the moral community. To begin with, membership in the moral community is relative to the capacity for taking moral responsibility. In other words, under ordinary circumstances there can be no membership in that community where the capacity for taking responsibility does not exist. In addition, it should be noted that most capacities for taking moral responsibility have to be *developed*, usually through the ordinary processes of socialization. Finally, it is a general moral imperative for any community that its structures and practices *foster* the development of capacities for responsible behavior wherever possible, and avoid the hindering of that development.

The moral community is, of course, an ideal. In pure form it exists only in the imagination. When the ideal is applied to actual communities, it must be tailored to the fact that some people's membership in the moral community is only partial—because of their limited capacity for morally responsible behavior. Children, for example, take on the capacities for full membership in the moral community slowly, and come to be treated as full members by degrees. We think of young children as full human beings because of their potential to develop into adults with full capacity for responsible action; they can be expected to develop their moral capacities in due season.

Other people have other kinds of limitations upon their capacity for responsible behavior. In cases of mental illness or senility, some areas of life may be severely marked by an incapacity for responsible behavior whereas other areas are not affected. In such cases, the individual is usually granted the rights of responsibility in areas in which capacity for exercising them exists. In areas where the capacity does not exist, responsibility is assigned to a proxy.

The situation of the mentally retarded is somewhat different both from that of children and that of the mentally ill or the senile. The capacities of the retarded child, like those of the normal child, develop, and with advances in behavioral techniques it is to be hoped that the developmental capacities of the retarded child may eventually be far greater. Even with the normal child, there may be a lag between the development of physical maturity and the development of emotional and moral maturity. In the retarded, this gap is far more pronounced and usually is never fully closed in some areas. The fact that this gap may be closed to some degree at a later point for the retarded, in terms of chronological age, raises the question of the proper age at which sterilization procedures should be carried out. This is an issue with which we will deal shortly. But for the moment, let us continue to consider the relationship between sterilization and the retarded person's entry into the moral community.

It has been noted that proxies may be used to make decisions in some areas for the mentally ill and the senile. Proxies may also be used for the retarded, for instance in the area of contracts and financial affairs. But one cannot have a sex life by proxy. Since an active sex life can have beneficial effects upon other aspects of the retarded person's existence, assisting the individual in developing affectionate cooperation with another person, and the responsibilities that such relationships entail, it can be argued that sterilization encourages participation in the moral community in at least some respects. Although sterilization denies the retarded person participation in child rearing, it may open other doors, leading to a more "normal" life in other areas. If it can be shown that the retarded individual will be harmed by the experience of pregnancy and child bearing, or that the capacity for child rearing is lacking, then sterilization, by relieving the individual of stresses in one area of life, may make it possible to develop more fully in other areas. By removing all chance of incurring responsibilities for which the person is unequipped, the way might be opened for undertaking other responsibilities which the person does have the capacity to deal with. Thus, rather than doing violence to the retarded person's human dignity, sterilization could in some instances expand the possibilities of achieving it.

As we have seen, the argument presented above has been introduced, in abbreviated form, in some court opinions on the question of sterilization. Justice Holmes cited it in the Buck case, and it has been repeated in a number of others. Yet it has usually been cited as an *additional* argument, as if to give positive reinforcement to a decision that is primarily based on negative findings. In court decisions favoring sterilization, the fundamental argument has generally been based upon three other rationales, either singly or in combination. These include considerations of genetics, of the good of the state, and of capacity for parenthood.

It has been noted that the genetic rationale has passed out of favor with the waning of the eugenics movement. There are cases in which the likelihood of a genetically damaged child being produced can be medically established with a high degree of certainty—but these cases are rare, especially in terms of the mildly retarded. Nevertheless, a few things remain to be said on this matter. The North Carolina Supreme Court upheld the section of that state's statute calling for the involuntary sterilization of those persons likely to procreate children with "serious physical, mental, or nervous diseases or deficiencies." Several key aspects of this rationale require consideration.

First, the probability of the child being genetically handicapped must be considered. Every couple has some chance of begetting a defective child. For "normal" women over 35, the probability of having a child with Down's syndrome approaches 1 in 100. Two minimum criteria would thus seem appropriate. Since everyone has some chance of begetting a child with a genetic defect, it must be known that there is a genetic condition likely to produce such a child. Because many mental illnesses and many kinds of mental retardation are not known to be genetically based, the number of cases which would meet this criterion is drastically narrowed. Indeed, it might be reasonable to require that the probability of producing a defective child be at least equivalent to the likelihood of such an outcome in a normal person with a monogenic recessive disorder. This probability will vary with the severity of the defect.

In making use of the genetic rationale, it is also suggested that other, less drastic alternatives should be considered. For some genetic defects, amniocentesis and selective abortion of defective fetuses is possible. If a person is capable of being a competent parent, these procedures would be less restrictive than sterilization. Moreover, if the person in question suffers such a genetic defect herself or himself, and is still capable of being a competent parent, then the defect is probably not serious enough to justify sterilization.

In court decisions, the genetic rationale is often intertwined with considerations as to a possible burden to the state, which would be called upon to care for a defective child. The burden to the state might also arise in cases where the parents were incapable of caring for the child. Here, general social interests are cited, interests that go beyond either the potential retarded parents or their possible children. If children might have genetic mental or physical defects, or parents might require special supportive services, it is argued, there will be additional burdens on society in providing necessary care. However, since these burdens would be primarily financial, they do not seem by themselves to justify sterilization. Fundamental rights cannot justifiably be abrogated merely because respecting them involves expense. At the least, the expense involved would have to be such as to significantly decrease the ability of the state to carry out other appropriate functions.

It is the third rationale, concerning the retarded person's ability to serve as a parent, that is the most complex and in some ways the most valid. It is frequently claimed that the state's interest in preventing harm to particular children is compelling. This reasoning, by itself, seems unsound to many. Prior to conception, no particular child can be identified. That is, there is no particular individual who can be harmed. More importantly, few children who were born would be harmed. They would not have their lives made worse, because had their parents been sterilized, they would not exist. Children can be harmed, from one point of view, only if they are brought into existence and their lives are so miserable that they are worse than nonexistence. Such cases are rare.

This argument, however, does not eliminate all rationales based upon the well-being of possible children. The state has obligations to provide all citizens a minimum level of welfare and equality of opportunity. If the state has an obligation to provide these benefits, then it may reasonably ensure that future citizens are capable of attaining and taking advantage of them. To quote once again from the opinion of the Oregon Court of Appeals:

> The state's concern for the welfare of its citizenry extends to future generations and when there is overwhelming evidence . . . that a potential parent will be unable to provide a proper environment for a child because of his own mental illness or mental retardation, the state has sufficient interest to order sterilization.

This opinion involves a balancing of the rights of the parents against the rights of the offspring. J. R. Kramer has written of the "right not to be mentally retarded."[1] Although it is true that genetic risk of retardation accounts for only a

[1]J. R. Kramer, "The Right Not to be Mentally Retarded," in M. Kindred, J. Cohen, D. Penrod, and T. Shaffer, eds., *The Mentally Retarded Citizen and the Law* (New York: Free Press, 1976).

fraction of all cases of retardation, it is also true that there is a significantly greater probability of retardation among offspring of retarded than of nonretarded parents. Thus, retarded parents who choose to have children would be opting for a significantly increased probability of violating their children's "right not to be retarded," to use Kramer's phrase.

In addition, the kinds of environmental variables which are most commonly associated with retardation—such as inadequate diet, lead poisoning, and so on—are more likely to occur inadvertently when the parents are handicapped themselves. It should also be noted that it is generally conceded that intellectual development is significantly affected by early language modeling. Retarded parents would unquestionably be less able to provide language and cognitive models that are as adequate as those provided by nonhandicapped parents. All of these considerations must be borne in mind when balancing the rights of their children. The question that remains is whether the potential inadequacies mentioned here are so great as to render a given parent actually incompetent.

The most difficult aspect of the parental-incompetence rationale, of course, is determining the incompetence. There are few clear sociological criteria for being a competent parent. Even among people of average intelligence, it is often difficult to judge in advance whether or not a given individual will be a competent parent. What is more, there is a tendency to go beyond the question of competence *per se* and to inject the terms "good" and "bad" into this debate. Thus, it may be noted that some people of high intelligence turn out to be hostile and neglectful parents, whereas others of much less intellectual ability make exceptionally nurturing and caring parents. What is more, because of the complexity of human personality interactions, the same person may be a "good" parent to one child and a "bad" parent to another. Finally, it is easier to identify things that are "bad" in a parent than things that are "good." Thus, a parent who beats or abuses a child is quite clearly a "bad" parent. But what are we to make, for instance, of the father who insists upon taking his son to a baseball game when the boy would rather go to the ballet with his mother and sister?

It seems necessary, therefore, to remove value judgments concerning good and bad from the debate, and to try to discover some criteria that are more objective. It is easier to do this negatively than positively; that is, to look for evidence of incompetence rather than competence. Approached in this way, the problem does admit of some possible solutions. For instance, in one of the cases we have examined, evidence was introduced that the young woman for whom sterilization was being sought had difficulty in controlling her bladder and bowels, and that she did not understand menstruation. Since one of the basic responsibilities of a parent is to teach children to control their bladder and bowels, and to assist them in understanding their bodily functions, it seems quite clear that this particular young woman would be an incompetent parent. A parent must, on a broader scale, consider and make judgments concerning a child's medical welfare. If a person is incapable of making such judgments for himself, then he or she is clearly incapable of making them for others.

It also seems reasonable to state that if a person cannot protect himself or manage his affairs, he is incapable of being a competent parent. A parent is a legal guardian of his children, but one who requires a legal guardian himself is incapable of being a legal guardian of others. Although the factual criteria are disputable in such matters, one writer has stated that parents with IQs of less than 55 or 60 are seldom able to provide proper care of children. Generally, the capacities for managing one's own affairs so overlap those of caring for children that it is doubtful that many persons who lack the former capacity will nonetheless possess the latter.

It was suggested that there were six negative characteristics which would indicate a lack of competence to be a parent: (1) lack of language; (2) pervasive reality distortion; (3) persistent malevolence toward a child; (4) inconsistency in value system; (5) inability to communicate essential survival information, or to act as a model for a child; (6) inability to establish interpersonal relationships. This list of negative characteristics was strongly challenged by some members of the group, however, on the ground that such criteria might be applied without first having made sufficient efforts to teach the mildly retarded to function more adequately in these various areas. Second, it was pointed out that many so-called normal parents may also be deficient in one or more of these areas. One member of the group suggested that a mild degree of malevolence toward one's children was a universal phenomenon. Questions were also raised in regard to retarded persons who exhibit other of these characteristics to only a mild degree. This situation is particularly likely to occur with the mildly retarded—the very people with whom we are most concerned. As we have noted throughout this book, the closer a retarded person comes to the borderline between being retarded and nonretarded, the more difficult it becomes to make hard and fast judgments. For instance, some mild degree of reality distortion or inconsistency in value systems might not rule out a capability for parenthood. Indeed, these defects may be found in a considerable number of "normal" parents whose right to children is never brought into question. Some would argue that this fact alone militates against depriving the retarded of the right to be a parent. For there is a clear injustice in the fact that the parent who is adjudged "normal" is sometimes able to "get away with" a number of defects in parenting capability, whereas the retarded person, simply because he or she is labeled retarded, is liable to the instigation of sterilization procedures.

Another factor that must be taken into consideration is that parental functions are often shared by a couple. If one parent lacks the competence to perform certain parental tasks, the other parent may be capable of carrying them out. Consequently, in considering competence to be a parent, it may be inappropriate to focus exclusively on the capabilities of the mentally incompetent person while ignoring the possible competence of the partner. On the other hand, given the high incidence of divorce, as well as the possibility of premature death or the incapacitation of the partner, it may be unwise to put too much faith in the continued presence of the mentally competent partner—at least without mandating that in the event of divorce or separation, the competent parent receive custody of any children.

In addition to the possible presence of at least one competent parent, the availability of support services for the mildly retarded must be taken into account. If it is possible for caseworkers to visit the home of the retarded person on a regular basis to assist in problems that may develop in caring for a child, does such outside help give us cause to classify a person who might otherwise be considered an incompetent parent as competent under these assisted circumstances?

There are several problems here. First, the availability of such assistance varies not only from state to state, but sometimes even from community to community within a state. Obviously, therefore, the particular town or city or state in which the retarded person lives becomes important. Assuming that support services do exist in a given community, would it then be necessary to require the retarded parent to seek permission to move to another community? If so, then the right to be a parent would be contingent upon an abridgment of the right to choose where one lives.

But even more importantly, how much assistance might the retarded parent require? There are those who argue that such parents should be given as much help as they need. Yet there are situations in which "sufficient" help might involve the services of a considerable number of public servants, dealing with separate problems that might arise in psychiatric, medical, financial, or other areas. Can such extensive assistance be justified? Here the state's responsibility for assuring the welfare of its citizens comes into conflict with budgetary and political exigencies. When the budgets for public schools for the children of "normal" citizens are being cut back, the services for retarded parents and children invariably enter into the political equation. And legislators are bound to ask the same basic question: "Why should the retarded be allowed to have children if they cannot care for them without the help of public funded programs?" Indeed it is possible that overall funding for the care of the retarded could be put in jeopardy in some states. Political trade-offs can occur in which some legislators agree to vote for increased aid for the retarded only if other legislators will support involuntary-sterilization statutes. Thus, whereas support services may in some cases make it possible for a mildly retarded individual to achieve competency as a parent, the provision of such services is not a simple matter.

In concluding this chapter, let us return to the matter of fundamental human rights. The United Nations Declaration of Human Rights states that "Men and women of full age . . . have the right to marry and found a family." The right to marry is not directly threatened by sterilization, although being sterilized may indirectly affect one's prospects of marriage. However, sterilization does directly affect one's right to found a family. The United Nations World Population Plan of Action declares, "All couples and individuals have the basic right to decide freely and responsibly the number and spacing of their children." This right subsumes three distinct rights: (1) to determine the number of children one has, (2) to decide to rear children, and (3) to decide to beget genetic offspring. These rights are obviously not one and the same. A law prohibiting having more than three children does not prohibit rearing or begetting some children. Similarly, people may be forbidden to beget but permitted to rear children, or forbidden to rear but permitted to beget them.

Nor are these three rights with respect to procreation of equal value. The right to determine the number of children one has cannot exist without the right to either beget or rear children. For various complex reasons, especially in common-law countries, there has been a historical emphasis upon genetic offspring—thus making it seem as though the right to beget children is more important than the right to rear them. However, when the act of merely begetting children is contrasted with the shared love and experiences involved in raising them, it can be argued that the right to rear children is of a higher order. But even if the right to beget children is of less value than the right to rear them, it remains a fundamental right. The United States Supreme Court has recognized it to be such, in holding that the right of privacy entails a right of the individual to "be free from unwarranted governmental intrusion into matters so fundamentally affecting a person as the decision whether to bear or beget a child." This opinion was not issued in respect to a sterilization case, however, and some would claim that it is the *capacity* to be parents that has been denied to retarded persons, rather than the *right*, and that the capacity was denied by nature rather than by the courts.

Sterilization, however, does directly affect the right to *beget* children; moreover, because it involves an invasion of the body, it also pertains to the fundamental right of bodily integrity. Sterilization does not, however, necessarily pertain to the right to rear children, since sterile persons might still adopt or rear children. Nevertheless, the right of the mentally retarded to *rear* children is often, as we have seen, a primary consideration in their sterilization. The right to determine the number of children one has is not very pertinent in this present context, since the issue is usually whether the retarded should have (beget or rear) any children at all.

To prevent the retarded from either begetting or rearing children thus deprives them of the two most important of the fundamental rights of procreation set forth by the United Nations. Two aspects of the United Nations declarations require a closer look, however. The phrase "freely and responsibly" is used in stating the "basic right to decide . . . the number and spacing of their children." If these words were removed, then the "basic right" would become unequivocal. Indeed, if the word "freely" were retained and the word "responsibly" removed, the declaration would be unequivocal. But although one may hope that freedom and responsibility go hand in hand, they do not necessarily do so. The free person may sometimes behave irresponsibly, and since what one person defines as responsible behavior may be defined as irresponsible by someone else, the use of the word "responsibly" in the United Nations statement introduces the possibility of both ethical and legal loopholes. Thus, since the entire question of the competence of the mentally retarded to be parents revolves around their ability to act with reasonable responsibility in respect to their children, it can be argued that if a person is determined to be incapable of such responsible behavior, then to deprive him or her of the right to beget or rear children does not in fact abrogate a fundamental right as it is stated by the United Nations. Of course, it may also be argued that the United Nations statement is badly framed, and that a fundamental right to beget and raise children does exist regardless of the inconsistencies present in this particular statement of that right.

But there is another phrase in the United Nations Declaration of Human Rights that is perhaps of even greater importance in considering the rights of the retarded to have children. The declaration states, *"Men and women of full age* . . . have the right to marry and found a family." The reference to "full age" presumably refers to chronological age. Yet the retarded person's *mental* age characteristically lags behind his or her chronological age. The words "full age" in the United Nations declaration could therefore be viewed as another "loophole," indicating that the retarded might not be fully included in this statement of the fundamental rights of procreation.

But, on the other hand, these words call attention to a grave difficulty that is particularly germane to the court cases we have been discussing. In many of these cases, sterilization procedures have been instigated—and in some instances carried out—before the retarded individual concerned was of full legal age. To many of us, this seems especially unjust and unfair, on ethical, legal, and practical grounds. When a juvenile of "normal" intelligence commits even the most heinous crime—murder, for instance—he is immune from the full punishment that would be given an adult who had committed the same crime. It therefore seems both ethically and legally dubious to sterilize a juvenile involuntarily, when the only "crime" committed has been to engage in sexual relations.

Moreover, since the retarded develop mentally and socially more slowly than the average person, it is entirely possible that a retarded individual who at 16 would be adjudged incompetent to be a parent might develop sufficiently over the next five or six years as to become competent. Thus, sterilizations that are carried out when the retarded person is still chronologically a juvenile not only violate standard legal procedure when dealing with juveniles, but also are likely to be instigated on the basis of what might be called "insufficient evidence." The fact that the retarded person is not competent at 16 does *not* mean that he or she will never be competent—at least in respect to the mildly retarded. It may be that competence will not be achieved, but so long as the possibility of eventually achieving competence remains, involuntary sterilization, and the abrogation of fundamental rights that it entails, seems to some an extreme and uncalled-for step.

But if 16 seems far too young an age at which to carry out involuntary sterilization, at what age would the objections raised here cease to be significant? In discussing this question, a number of situations were cited in which mildly retarded individuals had been sterilized at ages over 18, but where the circumstances still seemed open to debate. It was generally agreed that many mildly retarded persons continue to develop into their early twenties; it was also generally agreed that in determining the likelihood of potential further development the matter could only be settled on a case-by-case basis.

If determinations are to be made on a case-by-case basis, it must of course be asked *who* is going to do the determining. In the court cases we have been examining, the conclusion that the individual was so retarded as to be unable to function as a parent has been arrived at on the basis of very different kinds of evidence from case to case. In one instance, the judge appears simply to have taken the mother's word at face value. In another case, the opinion of a court-appointed psychiatrist was given great weight. Sometimes the determination has been made by the director of an institution. We will be exploring this problem further in the next two chapters. But in terms of justice and fairness, it seems clear that the "opinion" of a parent, a court-appointed psychiatrist with no previous knowledge of the person involved, and an institutional director cannot be regarded as having equal value.

In this chapter we have presented some arguments supporting involuntary sterilization under certain circumstances.[2] The state's concern for the "welfare of future generations" when individuals appear incapable of caring for their potential offspring; the possibility of excessive financial strain on the state's resources; and, most importantly, the possibility that sterilization may allow a retarded individual to participate more fully in the moral community—all these are reasons for involuntary sterilization that must be seriously considered.[3]

But, on the other hand, we have seen a large number of objections raised to involuntary sterilization. These include the violation of fundamental rights; the inconsistent moral position taken by different courts in different states; the seemingly unfair outcomes of some of these cases, resulting in possibly unwarranted sterilizations in some situations and decisions against sterilization in other situations where it would seem more clearly warranted; the difficulty of determining what is in fact required to be a competent parent; the fact that the mildly retarded may continue to develop mentally into their early twenties; and the fact that the "evidence" introduced to support sterilization in given cases is often suspect.

Given the variety and scope of these objections, it might appear that the solution to the dilemmas presented by in-

[2]For further philosophical analysis of involuntary sterilization and the rights of the mentally retarded, see Chapter 10.

[3]Chapter 12 offers a philosophical argument in favor of involuntary sterilization.

voluntary sterilization could be best resolved through statutes which permit only *voluntary* sterilization. Indeed a number of states have been moving in precisely that direction in terms of legislative initiatives. Voluntary sterilization would prevent harm to "future generations" without inflicting capricious judgments on the retarded, and it would allow the retarded to participate more fully in the moral community on the basis of a decision they themselves have made rather than through the instrument of a decision that has been inflicted upon them. Or so it might seem. But the matter of "voluntary" sterilization of the retarded is not as simple or straightforward as it might appear to be. In fact, voluntary sterilization raises a whole new set of dilemmas, which we will examine in the next chapter.

CHAPTER 7

Voluntary Sterilization A Viable Alternative?

To do something voluntarily is to undertake it of one's own accord and by free choice, without being compelled or obligated to make that choice. In deciding to be sterilized, the individual must make that decision freely if it is to be considered voluntary. But since sterilization is something that is *done to one,* the individual must not only freely decide that he or she wishes it to be done, but also, in legal terms, give his or her *consent* that it be done.

In making a "free choice," the person of average intelligence may consider a number of elements, including what other people think ought to be done. It is assumed that because the average person has the capacity to weigh consequences and reason logically, he or she will in most cases be able to withstand pressures brought by others if they are unreasonable and to accede to such pressures only when they are seen to be reasonable. None of us, of course, is always able to do this. All of us—including those of highest intelligence—are at times unduly swayed by the opinions of those around us, some more than others. But, because a person of at least average intelligence is regarded as being autonomous, he or she is accorded the right to make mistakes and to make faulty decisions.

In respect to the mildly retarded, however, a very different situation arises. Because many of the mildly retarded have difficulty in understanding long-term consequences, their ability to understand fully the significance of sterilization is brought into question. If an individual does not comprehend the meaning of sterilization, then he or she cannot be said to have weighed the possibilities and come to a reasoned decision. In addition, the fact that the mildly retarded are more susceptible to coercion than the average person, and often strive to please others regardless of the consequences for themselves, makes it doubly important to make certain that they understand what they are asking when they "voluntarily" request sterilization.

As with involuntary sterilization, the response of the courts to these problems has been mixed. One United States federal court has declared that the mentally incompetent are incapable of consent to sterilization. Since this same court also held that no guardian could consent on behalf of the mentally incompetent, this decision limits the rights of the retarded in respect to procreation by depriving them of the option to decide to *prevent* procreation through sterilization.[1] However, some courts have found mentally retarded persons capable of consent to marriage and sexual intercourse. Since general

[1]In *Relf* v. *Matthews*, 403 F. Supp. 1235 (1976), the judge refused to approve new proposed regulations for voluntary sterilization because (1) the rule-making process was not followed; (2) he would not authorize guidelines contrary to state law; (3) the terms "therapeutic" and "nontherapeutic" were not defined; (4) HEW was not capable of monitoring to prevent abuse; (5) the regulations did not require physicians to certify that the patient had given informed consent; and (6) the regulations would not achieve uniformity because they incorporated various state laws. In *Relf* v. *Weinberger*, 565 F. 2d 772 (CADC 1977), the court of appeals dismissed the appeal as moot because HEW withdrew the proposed regulations. For excerpts from the text of *Relf* v. *Weinberger*, see Appendix (p. 209).

mental incompetence does not imply the absence of any *specific* capacity, it does not necessarily imply the inability to consent to sterilization—rather, one must consider a person's capacity with respect to that specific subject.

As sterilization is a medical procedure, the question involved concerns a person's ability to consent to a medical treatment. In the common law, medical intervention without a legally valid consent constitutes a battery. The underlying moral and legal premise is that a person has a right to control his or her body and is to be protected from unwanted and offensive contact. In United States law, a legally valid consent has the following elements: (1) It is voluntary; (2) information is provided about the procedure and its possible consequences, and about alternative procedures and their possible consequences; and (3) the person is capable of comprehending the information supplied. Without these conditions, assent may not be considered a deliberate choice indicating a person's true desires or will.

But whereas these conditions may seem straightforward, in actual practice complications may arise. Let us look at a hypothetical situation. A young woman is adjudged mentally incompetent. Her mother has been legally appointed her guardian. The mother feels that it would be in the best interests of her daughter to be sterilized, and the daughter agrees. The daughter then goes to a doctor and says, "I want to be sterilized." The problem here is, how does one know that the daughter really wants to be sterilized if she is incompetent? What does it mean to say that somebody is incompetent but "wants" to be sterilized? An incompetent person may "want" to live alone in his or her own apartment, but be denied that right because of his inability to care for himself. Other people involved—parents, guardians, doctors, welfare workers—decide they do not "want" him to live alone because of his incompetence. Yet, if he says he wants to be sterilized, the same people may put aside the matter of his incompetence because the sterilization is something that they also want. They may reason that if the person is incompetent to understand what is at stake, the person may also be incompetent to be a parent.

In terms of our hypothetical case, another element now comes into play. The doctor may agree with the mother and feel that it is best to have the daughter sterilized. It used to be that most sterilizations were carried out in institutions, but now the preponderance of them appear to be carried out by doctors in private practice. Many of these sterilizations are never reported in any way. If the doctor involved decides that the retarded person's statement that he or she wants to be sterilized is sufficient, then the operation will be carried out without further review. On the other hand, the doctor may refuse to act on the retarded person's request. In some cases, the doctor may refuse on moral grounds, feeling that the incompetent person does not understand the full consequences of sterilization and that it would be wrong to proceed. In other cases, the doctor might refuse simply out of fear of future malpractice suits. But whatever the reason for the refusal, the retarded person is denied the right to decide what to do with his or her own body.

Obviously, therefore, retarded individuals may find themselves in a double bind. On the one hand, if sterilization is carried out even though the individual does not comprehend its significance, a violation of the person's right to control his or her own body may be perpetrated. But refusal may constitute a similar violation, even if it is based on moral scruples. Refusal may cause some parents to go to court to get a legal decision concerning the sterilization of their children.

But, as we have seen, different courts have come to opposite conclusions concerning the ability of a retarded person to make a voluntary decision to be sterilized. The members of this research group also have differing opinions on the matter. Those of us who are particularly concerned that the retarded be granted as much autonomy as possible, and believe that sterilization can assist the retarded to live more successfully in society, are likely to be distressed by the denial of sterilization when it is voluntarily requested. Those of us who are particularly concerned with protecting the retarded from coercion and abuse may be more disturbed by the "voluntary" sterilizations that are carried out when the retarded person is obviously incapable of comprehending what the request means. All of us are struck by the irony that in some situations the retarded may be sterilized *involuntarily* whereas in others they may not be sterilized even *voluntarily*. It is interesting to note that there are those who favor involuntary sterilization but are opposed to voluntary sterilization, a position that may seem inconsistent but which is in fact consistently protective and paternalistic.

In general, however, just as there may be situations in which involuntary sterilization is morally defensible, there clearly exist situations in which the retarded ought to have recourse to voluntary sterilization. What remains to be determined are the kinds of safeguards which would establish with some certainty—if not beyond a shadow of a doubt—that the retarded person's decision is indeed voluntary.

To begin, let us look at how such safeguards might be employed within an institutional context. Proposals have been made for a committee to review the consent of the retarded to sterilization. Indeed, as a result of the Wyatt case, the Alabama Supreme Court has required such committee review for all residents of an institution. In institutions, the voluntariness of the retarded person's consent is often questionable. We have noted that in the past many involuntary sterilizations have been carried out in institutions because of the belief that the person could then be released to society. With involuntary sterilization being blocked in many states by court decisions, the emphasis has shifted to voluntary sterilization. But there may often be a tacit assumption on the part of the retarded person that sterilization is a necessary condition to release—which obviously would constitute a form of coercion. In addition, within an institution there are many persons who might influence or pressure inmates to request sterilization.

Various procedural elements are involved in proposals for committee review, but the main ones are that the review committee be independent—with no member of the committee being involved in the sterilization or employed at an institution of which the retarded person is a resident—and, second, that a lawyer represent the retarded person. Other elements involve standard procedural matters such as the right of notice and the right to cross-examination.

Review committees should assess whether the conditions of informed consent are met. In this regard, they should determine whether alternatives to sterilization have been explained to the person and whether he or she understands them. The alternatives include various forms of contraception, the possibilities of abortion, and the availability of supportive services in child rearing. This is an important point, since not even the Model Voluntary Sterilization Act proposed by the Association for Voluntary Sterilization in the United States provides for a review of the presentation of alternatives.

In the Wyatt case, the court also required the committee to determine whether a sterilization would be in the best interests of the person. Although some feel this requirement to be an important safeguard, there are arguments against it. As we have seen, courts have permitted involuntary sterilizations which are not in the best interests of the persons themselves but rather on the ground of the well-being of possible children. *If* the well-being of possible children is sufficient justification for involuntary sterilization, then certainly it is a sufficient justification for a person voluntarily deciding to be sterilized. Moreover, even a competent adult can legally and morally consent to sterilization for reasons other than his best interests. If a mentally incompetent person is found capable of valid consent to sterilization, there is no more reason to restrict his rationale for doing it than there would be for competent persons.

One difficulty with committee review is that the rather complicated procedures it involves might well deter even a mentally competent person from seeking sterilization. The complexity of the procedures is likely to make it difficult for a retarded person to follow them; an individual might comprehend the significance of sterilization but fail to understand the committee process, and thus be denied sterilization for failing to grasp procedural niceties. Nevertheless, in the institutional context, committee review seems a necessary safeguard. For the retarded who live in society, however, the advisability of committee review is open to question.

First, the difficulty of dealing with the procedures themselves must be reiterated. Second, the bureaucracy entailed in providing committee review for all cases arising in community practice would be cumbersome and difficult to administer. Moreover, within the context of society-at-large, some of the pressures upon the retarded to consent to sterilization may be mitigated. Undue influence may be exerted by the person's family or social workers, but the retarded person living in society has greater access to other opinions than he would in an institution, and the insidious connection between sterilization and release from an institution would not be in force.

There is an additional safeguard that operates in the noninstitutional area. Physicians are—and should be—legally liable for performing a sterilization without valid consent. The community physician has some assurance of voluntariness because the person comes to him. Yet the physician should also be aware that pressure may have been brought by the person's family or others. In questionable cases, therefore, a physician is likely to obtain a second opinion about the validity of a retarded person's consent. The fear of a malpractice suit, especially among physicians in the United States, should be sufficient to ensure that they would request a committee review, were it available, in cases in which the validity of a person's consent remained questionable. Thus, making committee review *available* to community physicians, but not *requiring* it, would seem likely to provide adequate safeguards for mentally retarded persons not confined to institutions without creating unnecessary impediments to sterilization.

The adequacy of this arrangement can be questioned, however. Although it is certainly true that concern about malpractice suits is growing—even dentists, for example, may be reluctant to extract a tooth from a retarded person without seeking the approval of a parent or guardian—many physicians have in the past simply accepted the word of parents or guardians for *involuntary* sterilizations, and there is no guarantee that when the retarded person himself makes the request any further examination of the situation will occur. Furthermore, even if a physician were to request a second opinion, it cannot be assumed that alternatives to sterilization will be fully explored or fully explained to the person requesting sterilization.

The matter of explaining alternative possibilities brings up another point. If alternatives *are* explained, and the retarded person seems incapable of comprehending them or of carrying out such an alternative as contraception, can that person be regarded as giving "informed" consent? Information may be provided to an individual without that person absorbing it; the person will *have been* informed but cannot be said *to be* informed. Both legally and ethically the person's consent would in such cases seem highly questionable.

Finally, there is a purely medical question to be considered. Techniques have now been perfected allowing vasectomies to be reversed in a majority of cases, should the man later wish to have children. Restoration of fertility is not always successful, but the possibility does exist. With women, however, sterilization is less easily reversed. Once the fallopian tubes have been tied, the chances of restoring fertility with a reverse operation are at present much less than for men who have undergone vasectomies. Thus special care should be taken when it is a woman who requests sterilization. Since far more retarded women than men undergo sterilization, the number of cases in which an extensive review would seem mandatory would be very large.

Our discussion of voluntary sterilization brings us, in a sense, full circle. All the themes that have occupied us during our study of the relationship between mental retardation and sterilization recur here in an especially clear light. Whereas involuntary sterilization introduces both ethical and legal issues that tend to complicate and obscure the basic question of how much autonomy the mildly retarded should or can be given, voluntary sterilization returns us squarely to the fundamental dilemma: To what extent can the mildly retarded be protected without infringing upon their human rights? How far can paternalism be carried without its becoming repressive? Does the mildly retarded person's right to freedom of choice carry more or less weight than society's responsibility to its citizenry as a whole, including those not yet born? By labeling a person as retarded do we succeed in protecting him from his own incapacities and the exploitation of others, or do we rob him of human dignity and prevent him from achieving the fullest use of the capacities that he does possess? How can we define mental competence in a way that will allow the retarded some freedom of choice while at the same time preventing them from taking on responsibilities which they are not capable of handling?

Throughout this book we have looked at these questions from many sides. We have not tried to provide ultimate answers, since we ourselves do not agree on what those answers should be. Indeed, if there is one point upon which a true consensus has been reached among us, it is that there cannot be ultimate or final answers to the problems we have been discussing. The way in which a society treats its retarded members is necessarily evolutionary. This is true not only because moral perspectives can shift in response to historical events, but also because our understanding of the workings of the human mind constantly develops and changes. We continue to discover new ways to assist individuals and groups in developing their capacities—just as we continue to discover ways in which to control and alter human behavior. These discoveries may, of course, be applied for good or for ill. In the coming decades, as psychological tools such as behavior-modification techniques, and medical tools such as gene manipulation continue to be developed, there will no doubt be new ethical and practical dilemmas to be faced.

For the moment, however, on the basis of the complex dialogues that have transpired during this study of mental retardation and sterilization, we would like to offer in our final chapter a few options for the future, suggestions for ways in which some of the dilemmas we have considered might be resolved to at least a modest extent.

CHAPTER 8

Options for the Future

In attempting to suggest some options for the future concerning the mildly retarded, we must begin by recognizing that many of the ethical issues raised in this book cannot be fully resolved. The debate between those who believe that the mildly retarded do differ behaviorally as a class, and therefore require paternalistic protection, and those who believe that the mildly retarded do not differ significantly enough from persons of normal intelligence to justify depriving them of rights accorded the average citizen will continue to be argued. This ongoing debate inevitably means that alternative practical approaches to dealing with the mildly retarded will remain in force involving, for instance, an emphasis on special educational programs in one community and on mainstreaming in another, depending upon the philosophy of the individuals in charge of such programs.

Some of those who participated in our discussions felt that our intentional emphasis upon the question of sterilization tended to obscure the need for *developing* responsibility in the retarded, and led to an undue concentration upon the matter of rights versus paternalistic protection for the retarded. Proponents of this point of view stress that all human beings, including the retarded, are capable of growth and learning. They feel that in many cases, particularly among the mildly retarded, a lack of competence may exist because no one has made sufficient effort to render the retarded competent through proper educational training. For instance, in one of the court cases under discussion, it was stated that the young woman involved had difficulty controlling her bowels and bladder and did not comprehend the meaning of her menstrual cycle. One participant noted that although this might be an accurate statement of fact, the question that remained to be asked was whether any professional efforts had been made to *teach* the young woman to deal with and understand these physical functions. It was further suggested that since sterilization was only in rare cases a matter of urgency, time could and should be devoted to training the retarded to be better potential parents, or, in cases where sterilization was voluntarily requested, to finding ways to help the retarded individual to understand what was involved.

It was pointed out that in recent years those working in the field have learned many different ways to communicate with persons who are quite substantially retarded. This is not a matter of asking a simple question and expecting a direct answer, but rather of explaining and demonstrating the components of a situation over a period of time, and allowing the retarded person to indicate a reaction in his or her own way. Proponents of such developmental training feel that in the past the emphasis has too often been on keeping the retarded, including the mildly retarded, from decision making, whereas the present trend is—or should be—the opposite: to marshal every skill at our command to teach the retarded how to make decisions, from the simplest choice of food or clothing to more complicated choices involved in social living.

But whereas all of us applaud such efforts and believe that they should be further expanded in the future, some of us are less optimistic than others about the results that may be expected. For this reason, it seems equally important to many of us to face the fact that many retarded persons are not at present competent and may not be even in the future. Thus the debate as to whether or not it can sometimes be of benefit to the mildly retarded to undergo sterilization will also continue. It should be emphasized that those on both sides of this debate take their stance on the basis of ethical considerations; it is not a matter of one approach being ethical and the other unethical. Rather there is a clash between two different ethics, one holding that sterilization can sometimes make it possible for the mildly retarded to enter more completely into the moral community, the other holding that sterilization is an abridgment of human rights, regardless of the good that may issue from it. The object of those on both sides of this question is to *help* the retarded, however different the results of the application of the two points of view may be.

Although these questions cannot be resolved to the satisfaction of all, there are certain areas of consensus among the members of this research group. One point upon which we are in agreement is the need for approaching the matter of sterilization on a case-by-case basis. The competence level among the mildly retarded varies too much from person to person, with some showing strengths in one area and others in another, for any across-the-board policy to be valid either ethically or practically. But to approach the matter of sterilization on a case-by-case basis is not in itself enough. Even if each case is to be considered individually, the conclusions that are reached may still be contradictory unless standard assessment procedures are developed.

One approach to developing a standard assessment procedure that has been suggested in the course of our study involves the use of three distinct assessment models in conjunction with one another. This *triangulation* of the assessment process involves the use of a *medical model*, a *social system model*, and a *pluralistic model*.

The medical model was developed in the field of medicine to assist in the comprehension of biological malfunctioning and disease processes such as measles, tuberculosis, or rheumatic fever. Although the medical model is a powerful conceptual tool for explaining and controlling biologically based illnesses, attempts to use it to explain nonmedical phenomena have been the source of much confusion in behavioral assessment.

The medical model identifies biological pathology through specifying symptoms. Since pathologies are defined by their symptoms, this model has also been termed a "deficit model." "Normal" remains a residual, undefined category consisting of those persons who do not have biological symptoms. The model assumes that pathological symptoms are caused by a biological condition. Because the biological organism of the human species is similar for all members of the species, sociocultural factors are not relevant to diagnosis when using a medical model. Tuberculosis, for instance, can be diagnosed without knowing what language the patient speaks or the nature of his or her cultural heritage. When using a medical model, we say that a person "is" tubercular or "has" measles. Cause-and-effect reasoning is appropriate to this model because the object is to seek biological causes for observed symptoms. Finally, within a medical model a pathology can exist but be unrecognized and undiagnosed. For example, a person could have tuberculosis and not be aware that he or she was ill.

Because hidden illnesses may exist, medical decision making is carried out according to a code which holds that it is a more serious error for a physician to dismiss an ill patient than to retain a well patient. This set of values stems from the assumption that pathological signs are produced by biological malfunctions which, if untreated, may endanger life itself. There is little harm in suspecting pathology in a person who later proves to have no pathology, whereas serious consequences may follow if a clinician fails to diagnose a pathological condition and treat it.

In respect to the mildly retarded, however, the medical model is insufficient and may indeed create difficulties. With serious or profound retardation, the incidence of biologically identifiable disturbances is quite high. But with the *mildly* retarded it is very small—as previously noted, the vast majority of the mildly retarded suffer from no identifiable biological defects. Thus, although there is good reason to *look for* such biological syndromes among the retarded in general, the likelihood of *finding* them among the mildly retarded is slight. This fact prevents the medical model from being a decisive indicator in assessing the competence of the mildly retarded. In addition, the fact that the medical code of values holds it a less serious error to retain a well person than to dismiss an ill one creates a cast of mind in which suspicion of retardation may all too easily lead to labeling a person as "possibly retarded." And here, of course, considerable harm can be caused. To suspect that a person may have appendicitis brings no stigma down upon the patient, regardless of whether or not the person actually does have appendicitis. But retardation does carry a stigma, and even to be "suspected" of being retarded can cause the individual great distress.

For these reasons, it is extremely important to look for other evidence, beyond that which can be provided by the medical model, before making an assessment of retardation. It is here that the other two components of this proposed triangulated assessment procedure come into play. The second side of the triangle is formed by the social system model. Sometimes called the social deviance model, it defines abnormality as behavior which violates social system norms. Yet it takes into account multiple definitions of normality, recognizing that each role in a social system has its own set of expectations. For example, the behavior expected of an individual who is playing first base on a softball team differs from that expected of the same person when taking the role of truck driver, which in turn differs from the behavior expected of that person in the role of husband. To judge whether a particular set of behaviors is "normal" or "abnormal" requires four kinds of information. We need to know the system in which the person is functioning, the role he or she is playing in the system at the time the judgment is being made about his or her behavior, the expectations which others in the system have for behavior of persons taking that role, and information concerning the person's actual behavior.

Norms for social systems are determined by political processes within the system. The dominant group in a system establishes the rules which govern behavior for various social roles, and thus these expectations make "deviants" of those who do not belong to the dominant culture. Definitions of behavior are both role bound and system bound, making it necessary to specify both the role and the system within which an assessment is being made. Since social deviance involves a judgment about specific behavior, and the political process defines what behavior is deviant, cause-and-effect reasoning is inappropriate when operating from a social system perspective—unlike the situation that exists with the medical model. Indeed, the diagnostic values within the social system model are the opposite of those which hold within the medical model. It is more serious to diagnose behavior as deviant than to overlook deviant behavior. The process of labeling deviance triggers institutional processes which tend to alter the manner in which the person is perceived and treated by other members of the system, and to move the individual away from "normal" roles.

To clarify the diagnostic-value issue, it is useful to distinguish four stages in the development of a deviant career. Stage 1 consists of the behavior of the individual prior to its being labeled as abnormal by someone in the system. Lemert refers to this stage as "primary deviation."[1] Stage 2 occurs when the behavior is labeled as abnormal by others in the social system. They may respond by attempting to normalize the deviant behavior through applying positive or negative sanctions. Stage 3 is reached when there is role reorganization within the system and the person exhibiting behavior defined

[1]E. M. Lemert, *Human Deviance, Social Problems and Social Control* (Englewood Cliffs, N. J.: Prentice-Hall, 1967).

as deviant is assigned to a deviant role—the role of mental retardate, learning disabled, emotionally disturbed, delinquent, and so forth. In more extreme cases, the person may be removed from any role in the social system. Such is the case when the school expels a student or a family places a child in an institution or a foster home. Stage 4 emerges when the individual defined as deviant internalizes the deviant role, comes to perceive the self as a deviant, and acts out the deviant expectations. At this point, secondary deviation is complete. Social roles have been reorganized in terms of the deviant definition and the individual has incorporated a deviant definition of the self.

A fundamental purpose of the assessment within a social system model is to *prevent* the development of deviant careers as evidenced in the movement from primary to secondary deviance. That is why it is more serious to label or diagnose behavior as deviant than to ignore nonnormative behavior. This viewpoint regards the possibility of precipitating movement from primary to secondary deviance, by labeling behavior as deviant, as having more negative consequences for the individual than those consequences which may devolve from nonlabeling. Obviously, not all members of our group agree with this viewpoint. But it should be remembered that this triangulated assessment technique is not being presented as the only way to approach the problem; rather, it is offered as an option open to further development and revision.

The third element in the triangulated assessment process is the pluralistic model, which has already been discussed in Chapter 3. In the pluralistic model, test scores for a particular child are viewed in the context of a person's sociocultural background. "Normal" is therefore defined as performance near the average for children who are from similar sociocultural backgrounds. "Subnormal" is defined as performance which is low when compared with other scores from members of the child's own sociocultural group. The pluralistic model assumes that all standardized tests measure learned behavior and that persons from similar sociocultural settings are roughly equal in the opportunity to learn, motivation to learn, and test experience. Those who are emotionally disturbed or physically disabled are detected by other means.

The use of three components in the triangulated assessment process offers additional safeguards against misdiagnosis, and at the same time helps to pinpoint the areas in which competence is less than adequate. Currently this process is being used experimentally in California with a sample of 2,100 children (700 black, 700 white, and 700 Hispanic) in the public school system. The fact that it has been designed for use with children rather than adults may limit its effectiveness in assessing the competence of retarded adults to serve as responsible parents or to comprehend the long-term consequences of sterilization. But it does point the way toward the kind of assessment process that is needed if the competence of retarded adults is to be accurately measured. One of the tasks that lies ahead of us in the field of mental retardation is the development of a standard assessment process that can be employed in respect to the competence of the mildly retarded to serve as parents or to make a reasoned judgment that they truly desire sterilization and comprehend its consequences.

The development of such a standard assessment process clearly will not be an easy task, given the variety of viewpoints held by those working in the field of mental retardation. For such a standard assessment process to be truly valid, it seems essential that it be hammered out through the kind of give-and-take that has been the hallmark of the conferences that led to this book. Not one of us is likely to be entirely satisfied with such an assessment process, but if it fairly reflects the diversity of viewpoints among those concerned with the rights of the mentally retarded and our responsibility toward them, a standardized assessment technique could go a long way toward resolving some of the debates that have been presented in these pages.

Just as the development of assessment techniques should be an effort carried out by a group representative of the various perspectives on mental retardation, so too must any actual assessment of any particular individual involve a diversity of viewpoints. The proposal for committee review outlined in the previous chapter would seem to serve this purpose. The safeguards built into committee review would help to protect the retarded person who seeks sterilization from coercion, making it more unlikely that unwarranted sterilizations might occur. Such committees seem essential in the institutional context, and, despite the difficulties, should be made available for the mildly retarded who live in the community, if they wish to take advantage of them.

Neither a standard assessment process for mildly retarded adults nor committee review can serve to entirely resolve the moral questions that have been raised here. Perhaps, in fact, these moral problems constitute a conundrum to which there is no final answer. It would unquestionably be helpful to have a new United States Supreme Court decision, a thorough and wide-ranging revision of the Buck case, in respect to the legal and ethical problems surrounding the sterilization issue. Such a fresh decision, based upon the greatly increased understanding of the retarded that has developed since Justice Holmes's influential opinion, could not be expected to answer all questions, but it would set a precedent that courts throughout the country, at every level, would have to take into consideration. Such a decision would at the very least serve to remove some of the inconsistency that currently exists in the rendering of sterilization decisions at the lower levels.

The difficulty in bringing a sterilization case before the Supreme Court, however, lies in finding a case in which the matters at issue are sufficiently broad-based. Narrowly based cases, turning on technical legal considerations, can have a constricting rather than a broadening influence. Indeed, lawyers concerned with the rights of the retarded have in some situations persuaded the parties involved not to appeal to the Supreme Court for exactly this reason. In addition, as we have seen, legality and morality do not always coincide. Thus, whereas a new Supreme Court decision could be extremely helpful in clarifying some of the problems involved, it seems certain that the issues debated in this book will continue to be a source of disagreement in the future. The complexity of these issues ensures that equally caring and perspicacious individuals will continue to find themselves in opposition on certain points. This fact may at times be a cause of frustration, but it should not be cause for anger or despair. What we are really debating are fundamental questions of human society in general: Where should the line be drawn between individual human rights and the responsibility of a society to maintain the common good? How can one respect the autonomy of individuals of restricted or limited judgment while still protecting them from abuse or exploitation? How does one weigh the value of a freedom gained against a capacity lost? What are the best psychological means of promoting autonomy and independence, and what trade-offs are likely to occur between promoting these and other salient values? Where should the burden of proof lie when paternalistic measures are taken with less than fully competent individuals—with those who intervene on behalf of the marginally competent, or with those whose competence is in question (or their advocates) to demonstrate that they should be allowed all of the societal rights and privileges accorded normal adults? These questions are fundamental not only to the rights of the retarded, but to the rights of all human beings in respect to countless legal and ethical dilemmas. If there were easy answers to these dilemmas we would all be, as individuals and as a species, other than we are.

PART II

Introduction

The papers comprising the chapters in Part II were all commissioned expressly for this project. All four were published in professional journals soon after the completion of the project, and large portions of the chapters in Part I are constructed from the facts and arguments presented in these papers. As mentioned in the Preface to this volume, we decided to include these papers following the main narrative because of their sustained philosophical arguments and the fuller details they provide on the central empirical, legal, and ethical aspects of care and treatment of the mildly mentally retarded. There is, therefore, some unavoidable repetition in the materials in both parts of this book.

These papers were selected not simply for the detailed background and arguments they provide, but also because each focuses on a somewhat different aspect of the overall subject. Travis Thompson's article, "Distinguishing Mentally Retarded Persons from Nonretarded: A Distinction that Makes a Difference," is written from a behavioral perspective, and makes a series of related points vigorously defending the appropriateness of distinguishing retarded persons from normals. It thus provides a grounding in empirical psychology for a normative claim advocating a form of paternalism to promote the "best interests" of the mildly mentally retarded.

Daniel Wikler's article builds on the foundation provided by Thompson. Whereas Thompson's analysis rests its normative claims on a set of empirical data, joined with ethical premises concerning what can best promote the interests of the retarded, Wikler, at the same time, undertakes a philosophical analysis of the concept of paternalism in the context of placing restrictions on the civil liberties of the retarded. Wikler thus examines what follows from the facts that the retarded differ from normal persons in their basic competences and that those differences may result in retarded persons doing harm to their own interests if they are allowed the full range of civil liberties accorded normal persons in our society.

The second pair of papers in Part II focuses directly on the issue of sterilization of the retarded. In "Voluntary and Involuntary Sterilization: The Legal Precedents," Michael Bayles provides a legal analysis of the precedents and the judicial reasoning that lay behind key decisions in the last several decades. Robert Neville, in "Sterilizing the Mildly Mentally Retarded without Their Consent: The Philosophical Arguments," offers a number of different considerations that might serve to justify sterilization of the retarded. A brief summary of each of the four papers follows.

In the opening chapter Thompson argues that a distinction can and should be made between retarded and nonretarded persons. The author suggests a number of behavioral features that serve to distinguish the capacities of the retarded from those of normals, chief among which is their lesser ability to anticipate long-term consequences of their actions. Arguing against those who hold that it is in the interest of retarded persons to "mainstream" them educationally and to "normalize" their social activities as much as possible, Thompson offers evidence in support of the claim that retarded persons stand to benefit more if they are treated with modern behavioral management methods.

Thompson and his adversaries agree that mildly-to-moderately retarded people living in the community are subject to exploitation. Whereas both groups seek to promote what they take to be the "best interests" of the retarded, they disagree on the question of what counts as "best interests" and how those interests are best served. Thompson openly acknowledges that a number of his arguments appear to fly in the face of present trends in approaching the rights of retarded citizens. Yet he maintains that those advocating precisely equal treatment in all respects for retarded persons are misguided, in spite of their good intentions.

The debate between Thompson and his adversaries involves a mix of facts and values. Can any empirical evidence settle the disagreement over which is in the best interests of the mildly mentally retarded—segregating them educationally or mainstreaming them? distinguishing them from normals in the provision of special services? allowing for sterilization with adequate procedural safeguards versus prohibiting all sterilizations of retarded persons? Thompson cites evidence in the literature of benefits that accrue to the retarded when they receive specialized educational, vocational, and other services. Insofar as such evidence shows that the retarded can learn faster, enjoy increased autonomy, and avoid exploitation as a result of receiving specialized services and special protection not afforded normal persons in society, the disagreement is a factual one, subject to confirmation or disconfirmation by empirical evidence. But as soon as it is asked whether these benefits outweigh the benefits to the retarded of treating them like fully normal persons in educational, vocational, and legal settings, the debate at once becomes one of values, not facts. If ensuring the rights of the retarded includes granting them the "right to fail," it is no simple matter to balance the benefits of being treated in a fully equal manner against the benefits of being protected against self-induced failure or exploitation by others.

In his discussion of sterilization of retarded persons and their right to procreate, Thompson reminds us that the rights of offspring need to be balanced against those of parents. He questions a social and legal policy that is only concerned with the rights of retarded parents and neglects the rights of their children. By broadening the context of the discussion about the rights of the retarded, Thompson places the issue of sterilization in a wider perspective. A staunch defender of the rights of the mentally retarded, Thompson holds that rights should not be granted to them unthinkingly, in isolation from the rights of others who stand to be affected. In concluding that "mild retardation involves a measurable set of behavioral dispositions, which can be expressed in terms of measurable overt competencies," Thompson not only urges that appropriate distinctions be made between retarded and normal persons. He is also prepared to draw the normative conclusion that such distinctions make a difference, one that ultimately serves to promote the best interests of the mentally retarded.

In "The Bright Man's Burden: On the Right of Mere Normals to Restrict the Civil Liberties of the Mildly Mentally Retarded," Wikler provides a philosophical analysis of paternalistic intervention into the lives of the mildly mentally retarded. His analysis begins with an analogy: Consider whether it would be justifiable for exceptionally gifted persons to restrict the liberties of persons of normal intelligence. Using this analogy, Wikler examines the moral importance of relative intellectual superiority, with the aim of illuminating our conception of the permissibility of limiting the mentally retarded in their exercise of rights and liberties.

Wikler begins by accepting certain premises that may be disputed by others. He assumes that demonstrable differences exist in mildly retarded persons competence to perform life tasks as compared with normal individuals—the very premise Thompson sought to provide evidence and arguments for. Wikler also believes it is likely that at least some mildly retarded persons would damage their own interests if granted full civil liberties, and that they would be protected from such harm if they were restricted. But returning to the analogy with which he began, Wikler observes that the fact that some retarded persons pose a threat to their own welfare is not by itself a sufficient reason to deny them the sorts of liberties enabling them to take such risks. Persons of normal intelligence may also pose a danger to their own interests, yet a widely accepted liberal principle demands that they not be treated paternalistically, but instead be allowed the freedom to act self-destructively, if they wish. The counterargument to this position is that the mildly retarded lack some basic abilities that normal persons have: the ability to make their own decisions; the capacity to understand what is at stake, to weigh the alternatives, and to take responsibility for the result.

Wikler conducts his philosophical analysis by questioning whether we would be inconsistent in urging limitations on the liberty of retarded persons while denying the right of exceptionally gifted persons to restrict the liberties of mere normals such as ourselves. He attempts to relieve this apparent inconsistency, in part by arguing that for important life tasks, the person of merely normal intelligence is fully on a par with the intellectually gifted person. There remains a significant moral issue, however: Does fairness require that we (normals) arrange conditions in society in such a way that the mildly mentally retarded would be in the same position to claim autonomy as those of normal and superior intelligence? Wikler ends by showing that the morality of paternalistic treatment of the mildly mentally retarded reduces to a question about distributive justice.

In the course of commenting on the key judicial decisions and statutes that bear on sterilization, Bayles analyzes the concept of consent used in the practice of both voluntary and involuntary sterilization. He calls to our attention the somewhat curious fact that the doctrine of "substituted consent" is sometimes used to classify sterilizations of the mentally incompetent as *voluntary*, even when it is the parent or guardian of the retarded person who actually grants the consent. Bayles outlines the relevant rights in this domain, chiefly those termed "rights with respect to procreation."

This account returns to a topic central to the two preceding chapters in this section: the notion of competency, both to grant consent for sterilization and to raise and nurture children. Bayles notes that psychologists and mental health workers do not agree about the psychological conditions or criteria of mental incompetence, and points out that these disagreements are ones both of fact and of value.

Bayles takes up briefly a procedural issue not explored in the other papers: the use of committees to review the consent of the mentally incompetent to sterilization. Problems peculiar to the institutional setting are raised in this connection. We should recall, however, that the population with which this book is concerned—the mildly mentally retarded—are much less likely to be institutionalized than those who suffer more severe forms of retardation. Indeed, according to most experts in this field, to place mildly retarded persons in institutions is to lessen their opportunities for gaining increased autonomy and independence.

In his discussion of the different legal rationales that have been used to justify sterilization, Bayles inquires whether those rationales can legitimately be used to override fundamental rights—in particular, fundamental rights with respect to procreation (to beget and rear children). Courts have upheld statutes providing for involuntary sterilization based on two general rationales: genetic well-being and parental incompetence. But under the substantive due process doctrine of the Constitution, states may infringe fundamental rights only if there is a compelling state interest for doing so and the least restrictive alternative is used. Bayles examines what those interests amount to, and just which alternatives open to the retarded are less restrictive than that of sterilization.

Although a legal analysis is useful for understanding what courts and legislatures have done in this and other areas where law and morality intersect, as we noted in Part I of this book, knowing how the law has spoken on any issue does not afford us a full picture of the relevant moral arguments and sound conclusions. Complementing Bayles's account of legal precedents and trends regarding sterilization is the final chapter by Neville, which goes more deeply into the philosophical arguments.

In his essay, Neville approaches the question of involuntary sterilization of the mildly mentally retarded by focusing on the notion of membership in the moral community, following the Kantian tradition. Neville explains this notion by observing that the dignity that should be accorded to each person as a human being consists in being regarded as a member of the moral community. The philosophical argument he constructs strives to show that far from it being the case that sterilizing mildly mentally retarded persons denies them their proper place in the moral community, the procedure (subject to certain conditions) actually enhances the dignity of the position of the retarded in the moral community.

Beginning with what he calls the "humble argument" for involuntary sterilization, Neville suggests that the procedure is in the best interest of certain mildly retarded persons. He advances a number of considerations in support of this position, noting that if such persons were not sterilized, they would have to be prevented from engaging in sexual activity or conditioned to homosexual or autoerotic sexual activity exclusively in order to avoid the untoward consequences of pregnancy. These include the possibility of trauma stemming from pregnancy itself, as well as the prospect of improper care for their children.

Turning to the deeper philosophical argument, Neville begins by urging that special care be taken to ensure the mildly retarded as full a membership in the moral community as possible. He goes on to characterize the moral community, noting that the idea of a moral community should be treated as an ideal, and that when applied to actual communities, it must be tailored to the fact that some people can enjoy only partial memberships because of their limited capacity for morally responsible behavior. With regard to the retarded, the capacity to make informed decisions about sterilization may not be present, for the same reasons that they lack the capacity for responsible behavior regarding pregnancy. Allowing for the permissibility of involuntary sterilization makes possible an active heterosexual life for the retarded, thereby enabling the moral community to foster the development of their capacity for responsible behavior.

The structure of Neville's argument requires him to address several "Who decides?" questions, including empirical, policy, and political aspects. He notes the importance of ensuring that the process of decision is self-critical and allows for opposition to be voiced as a corrective support when necessary. The chapter concludes by reiterating the basic philosophical principle underlying this point of view: a moral community has the social responsibility to foster capacities for morally responsible behavior. Invoking that principle, Neville holds that human dignity is enhanced when the mildly retarded are enabled to enjoy humane heterosexual relations. He is careful to insist, however, that the validity of involuntary-sterilization programs depends on the development of criteria and diagnostic skills sufficient to discriminate the proper category of people, that is, those who meet the conditions set out earlier for selecting appropriate candidates for sterilization. Neville ends by reminding us that some people need special help in exercising responsibility, so society has positive duties to develop the capacity for responsible moral behavior for all members of the moral community.

CHAPTER 9

Distinguishing Mentally Retarded Persons from Nonretarded

A Distinction That Makes a Difference

TRAVIS THOMPSON

Are there any real differences in the way persons labeled "retarded" and "nonretarded" behave? I think that there are such differences, and that in the aggregate they can be counted as deficits. These deficits make mildly retarded persons far more likely than nonretarded persons to be subject

This chapter was published soon after the completion of the project in the *Hastings Center Report* (June 1978).

TRAVIS THOMPSON • Department of Psychology, Elliott Hall, 75 East River Road, University of Minnesota, Minneapolis, Minnesota 55455.

to exploitation, to be denied needed services, and to make errors of judgment that will have adverse consequences for themselves and others.

However, many advocates of the retarded, who may or may not accept my position that there are behavioral differences, will argue that no legal distinctions should be made between the mildly retarded and nonretarded. One strong advocate of equal rights for the mentally retarded has asserted:

> They know and understand the consequences of what they do. They can explain to others what they intend to do. They act reasonably in their own interests, and it is morally right that they suffer the consequences of their own actions. The law has formulated another set of assumptions for people who do not fit this profile. Such people are "outlaws."[1]

If we take this statement literally, a great many retarded persons would be labeled "outlaws" in addition to being labeled "retarded," and would end up in serious legal troubles.

Nonetheless, the argument against distinguishing retarded from nonretarded persons is hardly an academic exercise. Stigmatization of the retarded and discrimination against them has had disastrous consequences,[2] and those who argue against making distinctions have several important points to make. First, such distinctions lead to segregation and violation of rights to which all citizens should have access. Second, specialized classes based on the diagnosis of such differences do not necessarily benefit mildly retarded chil-

[1]P. M. Wald, "Basic Personal and Civil Rights," in M. Kindred, J. Cohen, D. Penrod, and T. Schaffer, eds., *The Mentally Retarded Citizen and the Law* (New York: Free Press, 1976), p. 6.

[2]E. Goffman, *Asylums* (Chicago: Aldine, 1961); B. Blatt and F. Kaplan, *Christmas in Purgatory* (Boston: Allyn & Bacon, 1966); P. M. Wald, "Basic Personal and Civil Rights," in M. Kindred, J. Cohen, D. Penrod, and T. Schaffer, eds., *The Mentally Retarded Citizen and the Law* (New York: Free Press, 1976); M. S. Sargen, "Labeling and Classification," in M. Kindred, J. Cohen, D. Penrod, and T. Schaffer, eds., *The Mentally Retarded Citizen and the Law* (New York: Free Press, 1976).

dren; they may be just as well off being "mainstreamed" in regular school settings and other activities. Third, since all of us exhibit to some degree one or more of the deficits characteristic of mildly retarded persons, distinguishing them from the nonretarded is discriminatory and may constitute a violation of their rights to equal protection under the law.

In response to these arguments litigation has led to radically different interpretations of whether such distinctions can be made. Burt, in discussing one Pennsylvania ruling, argues that

> any state program that segregates mentally retarded citizens as such from others is highly suspect, and . . . the courts will require states to treat mentally retarded persons indistinguishably from others, except in ways that are both very limited and very clearly beneficial to the individual.[3]

According to Burt there are three important aspects to the argument: (1) that there are no actual behavioral differences between persons designated as retarded and those described as nonretarded; (2) that "segregation" is a relatively simple concept in which it is possible to demarcate segregated state programs; and (3) by implication, segregated state programs will be unconstitutional (and therefore not provided) unless they are clearly beneficial to the individual.

Actually, nearly all training and educational practices in some respect "segregate" the recipients of those services from others. Even when a student derives educational benefit from spending part of his school day in a special classroom or working with a tutor, "segregation," as characterized by the foregoing argument, is being practiced. In fact, one could argue that partial integration of the mildly retarded child might very well be more demeaning than total segregation in a separate school or classroom. It has been established that even when there is no explicit segregation of retarded children

[3]R. A. Burt, "Beyond the Right to Habilitation," in, M. Kindred, J. Cohen, D. Penrod, and T. Schaffer, eds., *The Mentally Retarded Citizen and the Law* pp. 425–426.

in "mainstreamed" classrooms, retarded youngsters apparently distinguish themselves from nonhandicapped peers to a greater degree than retarded children in segregated classrooms.[4] This observation is supported by the recent finding that 60 percent of mildly retarded adults feel retarded people should be educated in special classes in school.[5] It should be clear that this is not to argue against integration of services, but rather to emphasize the fallacy of suggesting that integration has uniformly favorable consequences, including leading the retarded person to view himself more favorably and as more, rather than less, like his nonhandicapped peers.

In exploring the consequences of segregated programs (in any degree) it is not a simple matter to judge whether or not such services are "beneficial." Some consequences of segregation may be positive such as rapid learning; whereas others may be negative, such as possible discrimination.

THE EVIDENCE FOR SPECIALIZED SERVICES

For many years retarded children were thought to profit from specialized educational programming in segregated classrooms.[6] However, the research in this area is far from clear. In fact, the best-controlled study designed to evaluate the relative efficacy of placing mildly retarded children in a special classroom instead of a regular classroom found no consistent pattern of academic advantage for placement in a special classroom.[7] However, it is important to bear two

[4]W. J. Cagelka and J. L. Tyler, "Efficacy of Special Class Placement," *Training School Bulletin* 67 (1970): 33–68.

[5]J. Gan, A. J. Tymchuk, and A. Nishihara, Mildly Retarded Adults: Their Attitudes toward Retardation; *Mental Retardation* 15 (1977): 5–9.

[6]W. J. Cagelka and J. L. Tyler, "Efficacy of Special Class Placement," *Training School Bulletin* 67 (1970): 33–68.

[7]H. Goldstein, J. W. Moss, and L. J. Jordan, *The Efficacy of Special Class Training on the Development of Mentally Retarded Children*, U. S. Office of Education, Cooperative Research Project 619 (Urbana: University of Illinois Press, 1965).

points in mind about this study. First, it was based on comparisons among children whose mean IQ was 85 and below, that is, borderline, not mildly retarded. This fact means that a significant proportion of these youngsters would today be classified as culturally disadvantaged, rather than retarded. Second, the population consisted of youngsters who were in first grade in 1938 and the study was based on four years of data. Clearly, the quality of educational technology 35 to 40 years ago was entirely different from that available today.

Numerous studies have established that mildly retarded children can learn much more rapidly and can achieve higher levels of proficiency using modern behavioral management methods.[8] In other words, it would not be surprising if no differences were found between mainstreamed and special education placement if inadequate teaching methods were used. The real point, however, is not whether children profit more from mainstreamed versus segregated education. The more germane issue is the provision of adequately trained staff, curriculum, and teaching methods. In the last analysis, to argue that retarded children "do just as well" in an integrated setting as in a specialized one seems to overlook the critical variable: the educational plan must be individualized and provide the necessary support service. When that is done, as has been demonstrated in Texas and Vermont, mildly retarded children profit under either educational setting.[9] In both instances, however, retarded children do require specialized services, which in the Pennsylvania court language "segregates" such children.

[8]S. Bijou, "Practical Implications of an Interactional Model of Child Development, " *Exceptional Children* 44 (1977): 6–15.

[9]A. Egner and B. J. Lates, "The Vermont Consulting Teacher Programs: Case Presentation," in C. A. Parker, ed., *Psychological Consultation: Helping Teachers Meet Special Needs* (Minneapolis: Leadership Training Institute/Special Education, 1975): M. J. Kaufman, J. A. Agard, and J. W. Vlasak, *Comprehensive Special Education in Texas: An Evaluation Report*, Special Report to the Assistant Commissioner for Special Education and Special Schools, Texas Education Agency, June 1973.

EXPLOITATION OF THE RETARDED

Many community and state agencies agree[10] that mildly-to-moderately retarded people living in the community are frequently exploited. Unfortunately, there are no systematic data available on the relative incidence of such exploitation among retarded and nonretarded persons. For example, the Minnesota Department of Public Welfare estimates that sexual, employment, and financial exploitation occurs among 15 to 30 percent of their clients living in the community. Other community agencies serving retarded women have indicated that the majority of their case load includes women who have been subject to sexual exploitation in some form, but none keep detailed records, apparently to protect the privacy of these women. This area badly needs careful investigation. If these estimates are at all accurate, retarded people clearly need protection. To adopt Clements's language, many retarded persons would, indeed, "take their knocks" in exercising their "right to fail" if they were not protected from such exploitation.[11]

THE ABILITY TO ANTICIPATE LONG-TERM CONSEQUENCES

It has commonly been asserted, and there is empirical support for the notion, that retarded persons have diminished

[10]Interviews with the Minnesota Departments of Welfare and Education, Hennepin and Ramsey Counties Welfare Departments, Hennepin County Prosecutors Office, The Legal Advocacy Project of Minneapolis, as well as several independent social service agencies indicated they keep no separate permanent records of exploitation of retarded persons. All persons consulted said sexual, financial, and employment exploitation are common, with most estimates varying from 15 to 30 percent of retarded persons, and some as high as 70 to 80 percent of retarded women.

[11]J. D. Clements, "Reactions to Paper by Robert A. Burt," in M. Kindred, J. Cohen, D. Penrod, and T. Schaffer, eds., *The Mentally Retarded Citizen and the Law* (New York: Free Press, 1976), p. 437.

ability to delay gratification.[12] For example, when given a choice between two rewarding outcomes, one immediate and small, a second delayed and much larger, retarded people tend to select the immediately rewarding outcome more consistently than nonretarded persons.[13] In practical terms the consequences of this tendency can be serious. In everyday living the choice is often between an immediate source of gratification (for example, going out with a boyfriend) and delayed adverse consequences (for example, the consequences of leaving an infant at home unattended).

It has been asserted that among "the most basic social needs or 'rights' . . . of men and women are the freedom to love, marry and procreate."[14] It is unlikely that anyone will question the rights of retarded persons to love and marry. However, in assessing the right to procreate, it is essential to recognize that one is balancing the parents' rights against those of the offspring. Indeed, 70 percent of mildly retarded adults feel they should have access to special marriage and family counseling designed to meet their needs, a finding that suggests that they are to some degree aware of the complex obligations and responsibilities of parenthood.[15]

[12]D. D. Kurtz and S. T. Neisworth, "Self-control Possibilities for Exceptional Children," *Exceptional Children* 42 (1976): 212–217; M. J. Mahoney and K. Mahoney, "Self-control Techniques with the Mentally Retarded," *Exceptional Children* 42 (1976): 338–339.

[13]W. Mischel and R. Metzner, "Preference for Delayed Reward as a Function of Age, Intelligence and Length of Delay Interval," *Journal of Abnormal and Social Psychology* 64 (1977): 425–432; D. A. Morena and A. J. Litrownik, "Self-concept in Educable Mentally Retarded and Emotionally Handicapped Children: Relationship between Behavioral and Self-report Indices and an Attempt at Modification," *Journal of Abnormal Child Psychology* 2 (1974): 281–292; L. R. Franzini, A. J. Litrownik, and M. A. Magy, "Reward Preference of TMR's, A Little Now or a Lot Later?" Paper presented at the Annual Meeting of the Western Psychological Association, Los Angeles, April 1976.

[14]P. M. Wald, "Basic Personal and Civil Rights," in M. Kindred, J. Cohen, D. Penrod, and T. Schaffer, eds., *The Mentally Retarded Citizen and the Law* (New York: Free Press, 1976), p. 6.

[15]J. Gan, A. T. Tymchuk, and A. Nishihara, "Mildly Retarded Adults: Their Attitudes toward Retardation," *Mental Retardation* 15 (1977): 5–9.

In a recent article the parent of a retarded daughter wrote:

> A retarded woman should have the right to enjoy social and sexual relations whenever she finds them suitable and desirable, as part of a full life. Like any unmarried woman, she would need, and we hope would want, to prevent pregnancy . . . A retarded woman who is pregnant and recognizes her condition soon enough has the option of abortion. But an unwanted pregnancy is legally more difficult to terminate after the first trimester. . . . Even if the pregnancy is discovered early, proceeding with the abortion may not be a straightforward matter. . . . Even if tests indicated an abnormality, a retarded mother might not be ready to consent to an abortion. . . . To the extent that she is able to comprehend such a proposal, what could be more devastating to her morale and feeling of self-worth?

She concludes,

> The optimal approach is surely to work out critical decisions jointly, balancing the child's degree of comprehension against the level of meaningful consent that is possible. . . . We are now seeking appropriate medical intervention that will guarantee our daughter's right to full protection against pregnancy that she needs and can get no other way. If anyone feels that this right must not be granted, let him or her prove that such a denial can in any way benefit our daughter.[16]

Others have written of "the right not to be mentally retarded."[17] Although genetic risk of retardation accounts for only a fraction of all cases of retardation,[18] it is nonetheless true that there is a significantly greater probability of retardation among offspring of retarded than nonretarded parents.

[16]N. Mills, "Our Daughter's Happiness Depends on Her Being Sterile," *The Exceptional Parent* 7 (1977): M2–M6.

[17]J. R. Kramer, "The Right Not To Be Mentally Retarded," in M. Kindred, J. Cohen, D. Penrod, and T. Schaffer, eds., *The Mentally Retarded Citizen and the Law* (New York: Free Press, 1976).

[18]I. Gottesman, "An Introduction to the Behavioral Genetics of Mental Retardation," in R. M. Allen, A. D. Cortazzo, and R. P. Toister, eds., *The Role of Genetics in Mental Retardation* (Miami: University of Miami Press, 1971); E. Reed, "Mental Retardation and Fertility," in I. Gottesman and E. Kimling, eds., *Differential Reproduction in Individuals with Mental and Physical Disorders. Social Biology* (suppl.) (Chicago: University of Chicago Press, 1971).

Thus, to use Kramer's expression, retarded parents who chose to have children would be opting for a significantly increased probability of violating their offspring's "right not to be retarded." Here again let me emphasize the discrepancy between factors influencing a retarded adult's immediate behavior and the long-term consequences of that behavior. Although a retarded couple may want a child today, the question remains: To what degree will they be willing to forgo a variety of immediate gratifications for the long-term benefit of the child?

In addition, the kinds of environmental variables that are most commonly associated with retardation, like inadequate diet and lead poisoning, are more likely to occur inadvertently when the parents are handicapped themselves. Even when the infant's native intellectual ability is within a normal range, it is generally conceded that intellectual development is significantly affected by early language modeling. It is unquestioned that retarded parents would be less able to provide adequate language and cognitive models than nonhandicapped parents. All these considerations must be borne in mind in balancing the rights of retarded parents to procreate against the rights of their children to a normal and healthy development.

Educational programs for retarded couples, homemaking assistance, and the like may all reduce the disadvantage the offspring of retarded parents are likely to suffer,[19] but these are hardly guarantees of equal protection for the children's rights. The recent report of the President's Committee on Retardation[20] gave extremely little attention to the rights of the children of retarded persons. Such analogies as "the poor and the physically handicapped can marry even though they are not self-supporting; alcoholics and drug addicts can marry

[19]W. Fotheringham, "The Concept of Social Competence as Applied to Marriage and Child Care," *Those Classified as Mentally Retarded, Canadian Medical Association Journal* 104 (1971): 814–815.

[20]M. Kindred, J. Cohen, D. Penrod, and T. Shaffer, eds., *The Mentally Retarded Citizen and the Law* (New York: Free Press, 1976).

even if they are not thought to be suitable parents,"[21] are of little comfort to the children involved. If society has erred in permitting some neglectful parents to procreate, it obviously does not follow that our social and legal systems should do so with others. The point is not that marriage should be barred for retarded persons nor that involuntary sterilization should be encouraged. A social and legal policy that is only concerned with the rights of retarded parents and neglects the rights of their children is, however, questionable. There are other alternatives, such as more adequate means of birth control, and in the instance of parents proven clearly neglectful, foster placement of the children and possible sterilization of grossly neglectful parents.

THE CONTINUOUS NATURE OF BEHAVIORAL DEFICITS

Since we all possess, to some degree, characteristics similar to mildly retarded persons (for example, limited ability to anticipate future consequences of current decisions), some have suggested that it makes no sense to distinguish mildly retarded persons from nonretarded people. However, the scientific literature is replete with examples of biological aberrations having multiple manifestations, which exist on a continuum, but one on which at some point it is generally conceded that special attention or intervention is required. For example, there are gradations of diabetes, many of which go undetected or untreated. However, at some point, dizziness, shock reactions, coma, retinal degeneration, and gangrene occur. It is ludicrous to suggest that because a disorder of the pancreas is continuous rather than discontinuous, specialists in internal medicine would fail, at some point, to make

[21]P. M. Wald, "Basic Personal and Civil Rights," in M. Kindred, J. Cohen, D. Penrod, and T. Schaffer, eds., *The Mentally Retarded Citizen and the Law* (New York: Free Press, 1976).

the decision that specialized diets and/or medications are required. The fact that retardation is multifaceted and continuous is irrelevant to the fact that statistically the combined deficits of many mildly retarded persons render them sufficiently disadvantaged that they require certain protections for themselves and others, especially their potential offspring.

BROAD GUIDELINES FOR PROTECTION OF RIGHTS

The tenor of the foregoing discussion could lead to the conclusion that I am arguing for segregation of the retarded, limitations on their marital rights, and involuntary sterilization. Nothing could be further from the truth.

The solution to my disagreement with many advocates for the retarded lies in acknowledging the significant probability that many retarded people have limited competences and in providing broad guidelines to protect both them and others from their sometimes less-than-competent actions. Let me give an example or two to illustrate the concept. A mildly retarded person who has limited understanding of financial matters (understanding denominations of money, interest, time payments) may be allowed to enter into simple agreements involving small amounts of money, such as purchasing items of everyday clothing, but could not enter into contracts involving substantial amounts of money, like purchasing a car or house, without proper representation. Similarly, a mildly retarded woman who seems to have little understanding of child health and child-rearing practices may be required to obtain practical training and demonstrate proficiency at a children's health center prior to pregnancy.

One might argue that all prospective parents would profit from such an experience, an assertion few would question. However, it is far less likely that a parent whose IQ is 130 would not know how to take a baby's temperature if it had a fever, or would not know enough to call the doctor if the baby is vomiting continually, than a parent whose IQ is 55 or 60. Thus, there is rational justification for specifying required prerequisite skills as a function of intellectual, cognitive, and adaptive functioning.

In the case of grossly neglectful parents, presumably the mildly retarded parent would be dealt with legally in the same way as any other neglectful parent. Removal of abused children, foster placement, and required birth control education would seem reasonable degrees of intrusiveness, commensurate with the welfare of the offspring. A neglectful mother who repeatedly becomes pregnant after the foregoing steps would presumably be the object of a sterilization hearing, as would a retarded man who impregnates his wife and/or other women and abuses the children. This degree of infringement on the rights of mildly retarded parents to procreate must be balanced against the needs of children to grow and prosper in good health and to avoid unnecessary retardation arising from neglect.

I am keenly aware that a number of my arguments appear to fly in the face of present trends in approaching the rights of retarded citizens. But I contend that those advocating precisely equal treatment in all respects for retarded persons are well intentioned, but misguided—misguided because mildly retarded people do differ in measurable behavioral ways. These differences place them at considerable educational, vocational, and social disadvantages unless they receive specialized educational, vocational, and other services. Moreover, certain behavioral deficiencies occur with sufficient frequency among retarded persons that social and legal mechanisms designed to evaluate minimal competences to enter into certain contracts and undertake parenthood can be justified as rational and not unduly intrusive, when conducted on a case-by-case basis. Finally, efforts to deny differences between retarded and nonretarded persons are misguided because they are based on the fallacious reasoning that since some features of retardation are shared by nonretarded people, it makes no sense to distinguish retarded from nonretarded people. Such an argument is as absurd as suggesting that since the concept of twilight is so vague, there is no difference between day and night. In short, mild retardation involves a measurable set of behavioral dispositions, which can be expressed in terms of measurable overt competences.

CHAPTER 10

The Bright Man's Burden

On the Right of Mere Normals to Restrict the Civil Liberties of the Mildly Mentally Retarded

DANIEL I. WIKLER

In many states, the mildly retarded must submit to the guidance of competent persons or authorities before making important decisions.[1] These include the decision to marry, to have children, to enter into financial contracts, and to live

This chapter was published under the title, "Paternalism and the Mildly Retarded," in *Philosophy and Public Affairs* (Summer 1979): 377–392. It is reprinted here with permission of the author and the editors of the journal.

[1]The term "guidance" is not strictly accurate in describing the relation of a legally incompetent person to his or her legal guardian. Technically, retarded

DANIEL I. WIKLER • Program in Medical Ethics, School of Medicine and Department of Philosophy, University of Wisconsin, Madison, Wisconsin 53711.

alone. Generally speaking, adults of normal intelligence may make these decisions without obtaining the consent of anyone, and they value this autonomy. When persons of normal intelligence, acting through the state, take custody of the retarded, they do not seek the consent of the retarded, who acquire protection but lose their legal rights. If we claim that relative intellectual superiority justifies restricting the liberties of the retarded, could not exceptionally gifted persons make the same claim concerning persons of normal intelligence? I propose to examine the moral importance of relative intellectual superiority, and to consider whether it can serve as adequate grounds for denying full citizenship to the mildly retarded.

THE CASE FOR RESTRICTING THE CIVIL LIBERTIES OF THE MENTALLY SUBNORMAL

The standard reason for denying full freedom of decision to the mildly retarded is the alleged danger to themselves and to others. Each of these grounds may be disputed. The latter is often recognized as dubious, and the former probably exaggerated.[2] One might even argue that the danger posed by the mildly retarded person to himself is less serious than that posed by a paternalistic bureaucracy endowed with broad

persons are (usually) denied the right to make the decisions at all; for example, contracts made by these persons are void, and marriages entered into by them may be annulled. The differences among these legal arrangements do not affect the present argument. See M. Kindred, "Guardianship and Limitations upon Capacity," in M. Kindred, J. Cohen, D. Penrod, and T. S. Shaffer, eds., *The Mentally Retarded Citizen and the Law* (New York: Free Press 1976), pp. 63–87.

[2]Partly because many persons labeled retarded are in fact not mentally deficient, having been mislabeled by inaccurate testing and sorting processes (see J. Mercer, *Labeling the Retarded* [Berkeley: University of California Press, 1973]); and partly because the wide range of support services available to many retarded persons enables them to function adequately on their own.

powers, questionable wisdom, and inconstant motivation. Still, it seems likely that there exist at least some mildly retarded persons who would in fact damage their own interests if given full civil liberties and who would be protected from this harm by restrictions.

In the liberal tradition, the expectation of doing harm to oneself is certainly part of any strong argument for a paternalistic denial of liberties (doing so merely to impose a benefit would be harder to defend).[3] Still, again within that tradition, an expectation is not itself sufficient to make a case for restrictions. Persons of normal intelligence may also pose a danger or risk to their own interests. They can make impulsive contracts, enter into disastrous marriages, and choose occupations in which they are likely to perform poorly. Despite these possibilities they insist on freedom of choice in such matters; not only freedom to make good choices but also freedom to fail. Although it is not absolute, a standard liberal principle allows us to do as we please as long as the interests of others are not unfairly threatened. The fact that we are about to act against our own interests is not (generally) enough excuse to restrict us.[4]

Thus, the fact that some retarded persons pose a threat to their own welfare is not in itself sufficient reason to deny them the liberty to do so. This denial derives from an exception clause in the liberal principle. Although it would be wrong to place restrictions on a normal person posing exactly the same threat to his own interests, restrictions on a retarded person would seem to be justified by his mental disability.

[3]See J. Feinberg, "Legal Paternalism," *Canadian Journal of Philosophy* 1 (1971): 105–124.

[4]It must be reemphasized that this claim is not absolute and that there will be occasions in which it is fair to restrict persons of normal intelligence out of concern for their own interests. But since normal persons claim a prima facie right to do as they please, why should not the mildly retarded also claim this right? Although our behavior toward normal persons is occasionally paternalistic, toward the mildly retarded it is routinely so.

Some persons of normal intelligence, however self-destructive, are capable of making their decisions on their own; they have the capacity to understand what is at stake, to weigh the alternatives, and to take responsibility for the result. The mildly retarded, however, by dint of their retardation, cannot. We normal people must decide for them, just as we must for the temporarily insane, the comatose, and others unable to reason.

Or so the argument goes. As it stands, it is vulnerable to criticism at several points. One is the vagueness of the concept of "retardation." "General" intelligence is not easily characterized, let alone tested and measured. And even so, the fact that a person has been labeled "retarded" through our social sorting mechanisms is by no means a sure guide to his intellectual abilities. But I do not want to press these objections here.[5] Rather, I want to examine the presupposition that there are but two possible statuses, however uncertain their boundary: one of impaired and one of unimpaired intellect, the one lacking a right to self-direction, the other possessing it. For even if we recognize an intellectual deficit in the mildly retarded person when compared to the person of normal ability, there is no obvious and compelling reason to attach such moral significance to it. The moderately retarded have this deficit when compared with the mildly re-

[5]The lack of attention to these points in the present paper is not meant to suggest that they are unimportant. Indeed, as recent case law has shown, they are themselves sufficient arguments against public policies which fail to distinguish among degrees of retardation, which rely solely on group IQ tests, and which fail to take into account the particular abilities and social resources a retarded individual may possess. Such policies thus extend the protection of the legal status of "retarded person" to people without regard to their real needs. More importantly, they also extend the burden of that status, stigmatizing the individual and legitimating the segregation and discrimination which have historically been the lot of those placed in this category. Thus one powerful argument for granting civil liberties to the mildly retarded is that such equal treatment helps to avoid stigmatization and its adverse consequences. This gain may offset the risks involved. The argument appeals to our concern for the retarded person's welfare, rather than to any right of self-direction, and it stands (or falls) independently of the issue addressed in this paper.

tarded; and the normal person might have the same when compared with the gifted.[6] We may recognize, then, an array of such cognitive statuses. Do these differences correspond to a large number of distinct moral statuses? If the average, now deemed "normal," is "impaired" from the point of view of those of higher intellectual status, are persons of average intelligence for this reason subject to a paternalistic denial of civil liberties?

It would seem that if the intellectual superiority of normal persons legitimates their controlling the decisions of the mildly retarded, the same difference in intellect would justify their being regulated by the gifted. Our right to self-direction, however, is a right to be free from constraint from any person whether of normal, subnormal, or high intelligence. It is supposed to hold even when our decisions are poor and when others happen to know better. We are in the position, then, of using relative intellectual superiority as our rationale for regulating the retarded, while rejecting the possibility of this same rationale being imposed upon us. Unless the apparent inconsistency is resolved, we shall have to either find new foundations for our paternalistic policy toward the mildly mentally handicapped or abandon it.

TWO CONCEPTIONS OF COMPETENCE

The inconsistency of claiming immunity from paternalism on the part of our superiors while claiming the right to impose it on our inferiors rests, I believe, upon a certain conception of mental capacity.[7] On this view, which I will call

[6]Robert Nozick poses a related question in his *Anarchy, State and Utopia* (New York: Basic Books, 1974). His concern is with a policy of "Utilitarianism for animals, Kantianism for people," in which beings of higher status may use beings of lower status as means and not as ends. The issue discussed in this essay concerns only behavior toward an individual for his own good, whether it is paternalist benevolence or respect for autonomy; but perhaps the latter is a particularly Kantian moral attitude. Nozick's own resolution, incidentally, seems open to the objections raised below.

relativism, mental capacity is an attribute admitting of "more" and "less." The mildly retarded have less capacity than normal persons who, in turn, are less endowed than gifted persons might be. No categorization of a group as "mentally impaired" makes sense, on this view, except when understood as relative to the perspective from some other level. Normal persons, those of average intellectual powers, are impaired relative to the gifted, and the mildly retarded are well-endowed relative to the severely retarded. Intelligence, like wealth, is open-ended. As there is no point at which one is "fully wealthy," only more so and even more so, no one can be "fully intelligent." We may be able to distinguish various levels of mental ability through tests, but any line drawn between mentally "impaired" and mentally "unimpaired" is arbitrary. The line could be drawn anywhere else on the scale with equal justification.

The point of this relativist view can be illustrated by reference to the specific components of what are thought to make up the retarded person's deficit. The mildly retarded person, according to one authority, is unable to think about and deal with more than one or two aspects of a complex situation.[8] He or she is unable to defer gratification so as to

[7]This conception of competence, and that which follows it below, have structural similarities to the "statistical" and the "pathological" models of normality, respectively, of Jane Mercer's *Labeling the Retarded* (Berkeley: University of California Press, 1973).

[8]Travis Thompson, in an address to the Behavior Control Group, Hastings Center, New York, 1977. Some of Thompson's observations were published in his article, "The Behavioral Perspective," *Hastings Center Report* 8 (June 1978): 29–32, which appears in this volume as Chapter 9. Thompson's claim that the mildly retarded have recognizable intellectual and behavioral deficits is quite controversial. One reason is that the faulty labeling process produces such a heterogeneous population within the social category of "retarded person" that few nontrivial general observations can be made; the present paper concerns those who are "really" retarded. Another reason is that admitting to group differences between the retarded and the rest of the populace is seen as a political act, legitimating and even causing unequal treatment in areas having little relation to such actual deficits as a retarded individual may have.

make choices most likely to be of benefit over the longest run, and to foresee long-term consequences of present acts. Similarly, he or she will be markedly less adept than a normal person in handling abstract concepts, and in making the kinds of judgments conducive to smooth social functioning.

The average or "normal" person does somewhat better at all of these tasks. But it is plain that normal performance could be improved. An exceptionally gifted individual may have the ability to consider nearly all the aspects of a very complex situation, to defer gratification as needed, to look far into the future, and to be at home with the loftiest of abstractions. "Normal," in this context, then, will mean no more than "average," and "unimpaired" simply means as good as most others.

Any definition of normality in mental capacity which is based upon IQ scores is susceptible to a relativist interpretation. According to the American Association of Mental Deficiency:

> A person's mental capacity usually is determined by reference to whether he has the ability to manage his affairs with ordinary or reasonable prudence, is of sound mind, has demonstrated rational understanding or intellectual comprehension, is capable of making a full deliberation of matters presented to him, has the mental capacity to make choices and to formulate requisite judgments about those choices, has demonstrated an ability to engage in meaningful intellectual process, has sufficient intellectual capacity to grasp concepts, or has substantial capacity to understand and appreciate the nature and the consequences of a specified matter or to give intelligent consent to a specified procedure.[9]

These criteria could not be met even by very bright men and women if we set high standards for "full deliberation" or "consent." Nor does this passage indicate why "ordinary or reasonable prudence" should be enough. On the relativist conception, there is nothing intrinsic to average status which earns its rights vis-à-vis its superiors that other levels will lack

[9]*Consent Handbook*, Special Publication No. 3 (Washington; D. C.: American Association on Mental Deficiency, 1977), p. 7.

vis-à-vis theirs. Average mental capacity, which normal persons conveniently label "full" capacity, is simply what happens to be typical for our species at this moment in its evolutionary history. On this view, there can be nothing to convince the gifted that normal capacity is "unimpaired" or "full." As a consequence, our liberal principle, that a person of unimpaired intellect must be free to place his welfare at risk if he so chooses, loses its apparent reasonableness.

The inconsistency could be resolved by abandoning our liberal principle. We could accept the rule that superiors may impose their paternalist guidance upon inferiors who may be mildly retarded, normal, or even bright persons, depending on the circumstances. It is not *immediately* clear that we do not accept this view now. As Nozick observes, we must reflect on our principles to determine whether they do in fact give such rights to superiors; the difference between such rules and the liberal principle cited above is not evident in our dealings with the retarded. We would be forced to choose between them in practice only if confronted by some race of supermen.

Ought we endorse this benevolent hierarchy? No definitive judgment on paternalism by the gifted can be made independently of a comprehensive moral theory. Still, some education of our intuitions might be in order. It is important not to confuse the value (to normal persons) of the advice proffered by those with superior minds with the propriety of that advice being imposed whether accepted or not. Many normal persons might consent to a regime in which the gifted made important decisions for them. Others, perhaps noting that the lives of the retarded have not been rendered blissful by the intervention of their intellectual superiors, might not. Does the relative intellectual inferiority of normal persons to the gifted exempt the former from the protection of the liberal principle? I presume not; there is little difference, in a given instance, between a gifted person better able to deduce future consequences of a present decision and a normal person who knows these consequences through access to the relevant information. Both know better what the future will bring than does a normal person lacking the genius or the data or both. The liberal principle restricts paternalism on the part of governments composed of normal persons who may know better; presumably it does the same for gifted persons who know better.

Any persisting intuition that the gifted would be justified in imposing their opinions on the nongifted might be a product of the following reasoning. The normal person is capable of understanding that the gifted person is more intelligent than he or she is; hence he or she would, if rational, accept advice from the gifted person; hence, any person of normal intelligence who did not consent to follow the prescriptions of the gifted would have to be suffering from mental disability. Were this true, then even normal persons would be suitable targets for paternalism under the liberal principle's "exception clause." Any nonoptimal decision would be taken as the product of an incompetent mind, and the liberal principle would have much less scope.

In any case, we can reject the benevolent hierarchy, save the liberal principle, and still keep our rationale for paternalist restriction of the retarded by countering the relativist view of mental capacity itself. To do so requires that "full" mental capacity be understood as a "range property,"[10] one which is possessed in equal measure by all who possess it. Such a conception requires us to determine a nonarbitrary threshold, so that all standing above it are equally endowed and all falling below it are unendowed. The point of the relativist argument is that there can be no such line when the property in question is general intelligence. We need not dispute this claim; rather, we may seek a different (though related) property which, unlike intelligence, has the bipolar structure we require. The idea involved is simple and familiar, and will already have occurred to the reader. Mental capacity ought

[10]J. Rawls, *A Theory of Justice*, (Cambridge: Harvard University Press, 1977) p. 508.

to be seen not as a matter of intellect, but of *competence*: intellect's power in meeting a challenge. A given challenge may be wholly and fully met by the use of a certain amount of intelligence, if the challenge is not too great. Although a person may have more intelligence than another, he will be no more competent at performing certain tasks; his added power is simply unused surplus. Those lacking enough intelligence for the task will be incompetent to perform it; whereas those having sufficient intelligence will be equally competent however great the difference in their intellectual levels.

We have, then, a nonrelative kind of mental impairment, at least as concerns tasks for which superior intelligence is of, at most, marginal additional advantage. There is a similar kind of threshold for other tasks. It will often be the case that, though added intelligence may increase the benefit to be derived from a given task or opportunity, a lesser talent is all that is needed to understand how to avoid harm. Geniuses may be no more adept than normal persons in determining the safest investments on the stock market, though they may be in a better position to get rich. The threshold here distinguishes those unable to comprehend and avoid the "downward" risks from those who can; and all in the latter category are equal in this respect. Relativism applies, in such a case, only to capacity for realizing "upward" gain.

This conception of mental impairment and competence seems to support some use of the liberal principle. In the case of challenges for which a given level of intelligence is wholly sufficient, persons of superior intelligence are not of superior competence. Hence, they could not use the principle's exception, which covers the case of impairment, to justify the assumption of decision-making power. The same will hold even for the second sort of challenge mentioned above, in which added intellect assists one only in realizing gain. For as we noticed in the first section, the strongest argument for paternalism applies when the aim is to protect from harm rather than to ensure a benefit. If a given level of intelligence is sufficient to avoid danger in a given task, those of greater intellect cannot use this principle to restrict a person's liberty in hopes of increasing his gain.[11]

If the foregoing is correct, we have shown the possibility, relative to certain sorts of tasks, of a threshold dividing the mentally impaired from those of full capacity and competence. If this is to help in justifying our restriction of civil liberties of the retarded, we need to show that the threshold happens to fall precisely at the level of intelligence just below what we consider normal. The relativist, we recall, finds no reason to suppose that the level of intelligence currently typical of our population is just the level of intelligence required to master the key tasks a person faces.[12] Without such assurance, it will continue to seem arbitrary to pick average mental capacity as that to which a general right to self-direction attaches.

There is a natural-sounding response to this query which, though mistaken, deserves mention. This is that our capacities are suited to our tasks because of natural selection. It would be pointless for the relativist to ask why it should be that we have just enough lung capacity to serve us in our typical pursuits, or why we have just enough blood cells to avoid fatigue most of the time. The answer in both cases, of course, is that neither is an accident. Both traits are admirable adaptations to our environment and its challenges. There is, with most such characteristics, a certain threshold below

[11]No general distinction between "benefit" and "harm" need be insisted upon here. The harms in question in this discussion can be enumerated: they are those visited upon people who engage in unwise exercise of those liberties denied to the mildly retarded. The seriousness of these harms (not "harms" in general) is what makes paternalism a plausible policy in the areas mentioned in the introduction.

[12]Different tasks, of course, require different levels of intellectual ability for their successful completion. Any adequate social policy of paternalism vis-à-vis the retarded will employ a notion of "selective competence" in which the retarded person is judged incompetent with respect to specific tasks and (perhaps) competent in other respects. The present, general argument rests on an assumption that many of the important liberties denied the mildly retarded require about the same level of intelligence. The argument does not apply to the liberties that do not.

which the organism is unable to thrive and above which additional increments do not aid in avoiding destruction. The same process which ensures that the average human will have just enough of the necessary physical capacities might be expected to shape his intellectual endowment.

However successful in explaining why we have the lung capacity we do, natural selection does not resolve the problem of mental competence. The complexity and difficulty of the challenges facing the intellect in modern society are largely reflections of society itself. The magnitude of that part of human intelligence which is inheritable was presumably fixed, however roughly, before the challenges which now typically occupy us in society were set. Evolution might have endowed us with the mental means to design and build shelter, or to distinguish poisonous berries from nutritive ones, but it cannot have been supple enough to set our abilities at precisely the level required to fill out Form 1040 of the Internal Revenue Service.

These reflections, however, do suggest what must be the correct reply to the relativist's query. The threshold of competence in our society falls at or just below the average, because, first, the level of difficulty involved in key life tasks is in large part socially determined; and, second, because society stands to gain by setting this level so as to render the average person competent.

The social component of a task like that of completing a tax form is obvious. We need not marvel at the invisible hand of evolution for making us bright enough to compute our own tax deductions; those who designed the form are charged with the responsibility of gearing its difficulty to the level of intelligence which evolution and environment happen to have provided. Importantly for our purposes, this social component is prominent in most of the decisions which are denied to the mildly retarded under laws restricting their civil liberties. For example, a person who enters into a financial contract assumes an obligation to fulfill his part of the bargain and forswears certain kinds of excuses for not doing so. If he is buying an appliance on the installment plan, he obligates himself to send in payments and cannot default because of inconvenience, second thoughts, or even moderate hardship. At the same time, there are certain excuses which he does not forswear; the safeguards represented by bankruptcy laws may be seen as part of this complex transaction. These socially defined characteristics of contracts set the level of intelligence needed to understand and assume responsibility for risk. Insufficient intellect will prevent a person from foreseeing the difficulties involved and thus cause the person to risk overextending himself. At the same time, however, the severity of the penalties is kept within certain limits by the bankruptcy laws and by consumer-interest laws.

Essentially conventional, these arrangements might have been different. Society might have instituted rules allowing persons to annul contracts if they proved inconvenient or if the contractor misjudged his resources at the time of bargaining. Similarly, the burden of a decision to procreate would have been lighter had custom not assigned to parents the responsibility for caring for their offspring. Under these conditions, persons whose mental powers are much weaker than the average would be competent to enter contracts, marry, and make other important decisions without regularly risking serious reverses which they could not predict and understand. The threshold of competence and mental impairment would be set that much lower.

If it is, in theory, within society's power to arrange itself so as to render the mildly retarded fully competent, why does it not do so? Mere prejudice, a society made up mostly of persons of normal intelligence concerned only for themselves, need not be the answer. There is considerable social utility, at least for normal persons, in setting the threshold about where it is. Contracts which are void when misunderstood or inconvenient would not facilitate the exchange of goods. An appliance seller hands over the product in exchange for a piece of paper because he believes that payment will follow. If such expectation were lacking, no one, regardless of competence, would have a way of obtaining appliances without cash. The value of contracts and other arrangements, the very ones subject to control in our paternalist restriction of the retarded, depends on their having features which make them hazardous to those with limited ability. Normal persons make the world safe for normality, but not necessarily safe for retardation.

The same holds true with respect to other abilities and capacities. The strength a person must have to be "unimpaired" is not set by biological limits but by the demands of society. It is, then, no surprise that those who design manual-gearshift mechanisms and who set the size of grocery bags manufacture products which presuppose something like the average amount of strength. The majority of normal persons in the society benefit (in a purely economic sense) by having the requirements this high. We could make do with levers and containers which even the very weak could handle; but these would undoubtedly be of less use to us. It is also worth noting that current practice sets the threshold for physical competence, and thus renders equal all those at or above the threshold. Those of average strength are just as competent as the very strong in moving gearshift levers; the advantages of exceptional strength lie in other, more esoteric pursuits. Increments of strength, like increments of intelligence, are important if they put one over the socially defined threshold of "full" or "unimpaired" performance. Superiority past that point counts much less, both for the individual's welfare and for our moral theorizing about him.

Of course, the average requirements, whether for intelligence or for physical strength, could also be set much higher than they presently are. A society designed by and for persons who are by present standards gifted would be a risk-laden environment for persons of merely normal intelligence. They would find themselves unable to understand the nature of the contracts and other social arrangements to which they would be parties, and probably would be branded incompetent. This seems, after all, to "find for," that is, decide the case in favor of, the relativist: the argument that is supposed to show that we may restrict the liberties of the mildly retarded would also show that the gifted have the right to impose restraints upon us—provided, however, that the environments in question also differ in relative difficulty.

Does this argument in fact undermine the standard grounds—need together with incompetence—for denying liberties to the retarded? Only if, as before, we insist that the gifted would not have the right to deny liberties to normal persons in the gifted society. Those who support our present treatment of the retarded on the basis of the liberal principle might wish to abandon this insistence, thereby removing any appearance of inconsistency in their approach to the two groups. But I do not think the liberal can abandon it. The intuition behind the liberal principle remains firm: we have a right to make unconstrained choices, assume risks, and even court disaster; and we have this right because of our rational faculty. Being placed in a demanding environment, such as a society designed for the gifted, does not diminish our intellectual endowment. To accept paternalistic treatment of normal persons in the gifted society because of the severity of the challenges would commit us to accept also paternalistic denial of liberty in our present society in those circumstances in which a normal person meets a strenuous challenge. Since this is exactly what the liberal rejects, he must refuse to endorse paternalistic treatment of the normal person by the gifted person.

The liberal should argue instead that the normal person who finds himself in a society created for the gifted would realize that his powers are inadequate for achieving an understanding and mastery of the tasks confronting him. He would, therefore, seek out guidance from a friendly gifted person; or if he did not, he would at least be in a position to assess the risks attendant on making his own decisions. Although, by hypothesis, he is incompetent to make many kinds of decisions that society requires him to make, he remains fully competent to recognize his limitations and to decide to seek help. On the liberal view, his intellectual powers will be sufficient to allow him to shoulder responsibility for what might happen, and this fact is enough to render a paternalistic denial of liberty to those of normal intelligence unjustified.

Again, however, the relativist has a response to the liberal. He can claim that humility, the disposition to recognize one's own limitations, emerges not with a given level of intelligence but with certain traits of character and temperament (indeed, it is such a trait). Besides, the retarded person is often capable of understanding the principle, "Seek guidance when you need it." His alleged problem is in knowing when it is needed;[13] and the same problem might well afflict the person of average intelligence who finds himself in the troubling environment of the society of the gifted. The notion that a right to self-direction attaches to those of a given level of intelligence, simply because of that mental ability and regardless of environmental circumstances, seems impossible to defend. Attempts to found such a moral right on the metaphysical properties of persons offer no help to average human beings (or retarded ones); for in these theories "person" is an ideal, the maximally rational reflective agent. As Dennett has argued, few if any human beings are "persons" in the sense which Kant and Rawls seem to require.[14] Human beings of average intellect, living in their own society, can insist on autonomy not because they are "persons" in this ideal sense but because, with respect to the challenges they have fashioned for themselves, they are nearly on a par with persons.

DISTRIBUTING THE BURDENS OF INCOMPETENCE

Before applying these conclusions to the moral issue of civil liberties for the retarded, it will be useful to review and summarize the arguments thus far presented. Restrictions on

[13]See Chapter 9.

[14]D. Dennett, "Conditions of Personhood," in A. Rorty, ed., *The Identities of Persons* (Berkeley: University of California Press, 1976), pp. 175–196.

the mildly retarded are usually justified by citing the dangers the person can inflict on himself. This justification, in turn, is thought to legitimate paternalistic intervention because the retarded person, being mentally deficient, does not have the right to self-direction claimed by the normal person. We may grant that many so-called retarded persons are in fact normal, and that many of those who are not normal are capable of living freely and independently without unacceptable risk to their welfare. The question which remains, then, is whether restrictions are defensible for those who are in fact retarded and who do seem likely to encounter trouble if granted full citizenship. If the right to take risks is to be denied the retarded by normal persons on the basis of the latter's intellectual superiority, one would think it legitimate for exceptionally gifted persons to do the same to normal persons. The right to self-direction claimed by normal persons, however, seems to be a claim of immunity against the paternalistic interventions even of those who are more gifted.

I have sought to relieve this apparent inconsistency, and to show that, for certain important tasks, the person of merely normal intelligence is fully the equal of his intellectual superior. But the moral issue is not yet settled. My argument, although showing that the threshold between mental incompetence and competence is not arbitrary,[15] also shows it to be set by society. As such, it could also be changed. Arrangements could be made to create the conditions under which the retarded would be in the same position to claim autonomy as those of normal and superior intelligence. We would need to show that fairness does not compel us to make these changes before we could regard the restriction of liberties of the retarded as justified.

There is no simple solution to the problem. We may say at once that society, through consumer laws, for example,

[15]The boundary is, of course, a vague one. The decision to draw the line at some precise point between average intelligence and severe retardation is arbitrary. What is nonarbitrary, according to my argument, is the drawing of the line at some point *below* the average rather than above it.

ought to make its institutions, customs, and practices as safe as possible insofar as it can do so without compromising their utility. To do so would serve to make the risks involved understandable to those with limited intelligence and hence in some matters give them the status of competent persons with a right to make their own decisions. To change society so that mild mental retardation would be no handicap in any of the tasks in question might reduce the economic and social value of the relevant practices, thereby shifting hardships from the retarded onto those of normal and high intelligence. I have no way of estimating the degree of hardship at stake. If it is substantial enough to seriously impede economic and social functioning, perhaps the majority, which consists of normal persons, would have no obligation to change present practices so radically. *Some* redistribution of burdens, however, is undoubtedly in order.

The fairness of denying civil liberties to the mildly retarded depends, then, on the legitimacy of giving higher priority to general social welfare than to doing what is necessary to achieve equal liberty for all. Given our concern that the mildly retarded not be pushed out into a dangerous world in which they may come to ruin, we have two choices. We may change the world so as to render it safer for all. Or we may refrain from allowing the retarded access to it. The morality of paternalism reduces to a question about distributive justice.

CHAPTER 11

Voluntary and Involuntary Sterilization

The Legal Precedents

MICHAEL D. BAYLES

Involuntary sterilization of the mentally incompetent has been seriously considered or practiced in the United States since Indiana adopted the first eugenic-sterilization statute in 1907. However, the practice did not become widespread until the Supreme Court upheld the constitutional validity of such statutes in 1927. The Court held that a Virginia statute did not violate the due process clause of the Fourteenth Amendment. In Justice Oliver Wendell Holmes's often-quoted words:

> We have seen more than once that the public welfare may call upon the best citizens for their lives. It would be strange if it could not call upon those who already sap the strength of

This Chapter was published soon after the completion of the project in the *Hastings Center Report (June 1978).*

MICHAEL D. BAYLES • Westminster Institute for Ethics and Human Values, Westminster College, London, Ontario, Canada N6G 2M2.

> the State for these lesser sacrifices, often not felt to be such by those concerned, in order to prevent our being swamped with incompetence. It is better for all the world, if instead of waiting to execute degenerate offspring for crime, or to let them starve for their imbecility, society can prevent those who are manifestly unfit from continuing their kind. The principle that sustains compulsory vaccination is broad enough to cover cutting the Fallopian tubes . . . . Three generations of imbeciles are enough.[1]

In the 1940s the Supreme Court's attitude shifted, possibly as a result of the Nazi venture into eugenic sterilization. In 1942 an Oklahoma statute was held unconstitutional as a violation of the equal-protection clause of the Fourteenth Amendment.[2] The Oklahoma statute also permitted sterilization of habitual offenders, and the Court could find no rationale in its including those guilty of larceny but excluding those guilty of embezzlement. Nonetheless, the earlier decision upholding the constitutionality of eugenic-sterilization statutes was not and has not been overruled.

In recent years, courts have ruled both for and against involuntary sterilization of the mentally incompetent. In 1974, in holding invalid Department of Health, Education and Welfare regulations for funding voluntary sterilizations of the mentally incompetent, Judge Gerhard Gesell claimed that no mentally incompetent person is capable of consenting to sterilization.[3] The Montana legislature passed a statute prohibiting involuntary sterilization of the mentally incompetent.[4] Yet, the Oregon Court of Appeals found that

> the state's concern for the welfare of its citizenry extends to future generations and when there is overwhelming evidence . . . that a potential parent will be unable to provide a proper environment for a child because of his own mental illness or mental retardation, the state has sufficient interest to order sterilization.

---

[1] *Buck* v. *Bell*, 274 U. S. 200, 207 (1927). See Appendix (p. 205) for text of this decision.

[2] *Skinner* v. *Oklahoma*, 316 U. S. 535 (1942).

[3] *Relf* v. *Weinberger*, 372 F. Supp. 1196 (D. D.C. 1974). See Appendix (p. 209) for text.

[4] Mont. Rev. Codes Ann. §69–6406 (Cum. Supp. 1977).

The North Carolina Supreme Court as well as a special three-member federal district court have upheld a statute providing for involuntary sterilization of those persons unable to care for children or likely to procreate children with "serious physical, mental, or nervous diseases or deficiencies."[6]

Against this background of recent, divergent actions by legislatures and courts, issues of sterilization of the mentally incompetent require ethical clarification and analysis.

RIGHTS WITH RESPECT TO PROCREATION

The United Nations Declaration of Human Rights states that "men and women of full age . . . have the right to marry and to found a family."[7] The right to marry is not directly threatened by sterilization, although being sterilized may indirectly affect one's prospects of marriage. However, sterilization does directly affect one's right to start a family. The United Nations World Population Plan of Action declares, "All couples and individuals have the basic right to decide freely and responsibly the number and spacing of their children. . . . "[8] This right is really three distinct rights: (1) to decide to rear children; (2) to decide to beget genetic offspring; and (3) to determine the number of children one will have. These rights are obviously not the same, but they are all based on the freedom to decide, and they encompass decisions both to have and not to have children. They may be called rights with respect to procreation.

Sterilization always pertains to the right to beget children. Because it involves an invasion of the body, it also pertains

[5]*Cook* v. *State*, 9 Or. App. 224, 495 P. 2d. 768, 771–72 (1972).

[6]N.C. Gen. Stat §35–43; In re Moore, 221 S.E.2d 307 (N.C. 1976); *North Carolina Assn. for Retarded Children* v. *North Carolina*, 420 F. Supp. 459 (M.D. N.C. 1976).

[7]In D. D. Raphael, ed., *Political Theory and the Rights of Man* (Bloomington: Indiana University Press, 1967), p. 145, Article 16(1).

[8]In *The Population Debate: Dimensions and Perspectives*, Papers of the World Population Conference, Bucharest, 1974, 2 vols. (New York: United Nations, 1975), I, 157, par. 14(f).

to the fundamental right of bodily integrity. It does not necessarily pertain to the right to rear children, since sterile persons might still adopt or rear children; however, the right of the mentally incompetent to rear children is often a primary consideration in their sterilization. The right to determine the number of children one has is not very pertinent in the present context, since usually the issue is whether the mentally incompetent should have (beget or rear) any children at all.

THE MENTALLY INCOMPETENT

It is difficult to formulate a general standard of who is mentally incompetent. Courts usually determine incompetence for a specific purpose, and the standards vary depending upon the purpose. For present purposes, the best legal standard is that for the appointment of a guardian, whether a person is "incapable of understanding and acting in the ordinary affairs of life."[9] The general legal standard of mental incompetence I use here is that a person is "incapable of protecting himself or properly managing his property or affairs,"[10] with emphasis upon the inability to provide self-protection.

Unfortunately, psychologists and mental health workers do not agree about the psychological conditions or criteria of mental incompetence. Both factual and value disagreements are involved. People with different values have different conceptions of what is needed to protect oneself. For example, some claim that the criterion that all people with an IQ below 70 are incompetent is too stringent, does not allow for individual variation, and uses the wrong basic measure. Moreover, it is now unpopular to make judgments about general mental incompetence; the emphasis is upon specific functional incompetence.

[9]39 Am. Jur. 2d Guardian and Ward Section 20, pp. 22–23 (1968).
[10]44 C.J.S. Insane Persons Section 11, p. 64 (1945).

VOLUNTARY STERILIZATION

Consent

A federal district court has declared that the mentally incompetent are incapable of consent to sterilization.[11] The court also held that no guardian can consent on behalf of the mentally incompetent. This decision limits the rights of the mentally incompetent with respect to procreation and deprives them of the option to decide not to procreate by being sterilized. However, some courts have found mentally retarded persons capable of consent to marriage, sexual intercourse, and contracts.[12]

Since general mental incompetence does not imply absence of any specific capacity, it does not imply the inability to consent to sterilization. One must consider a person's capacity with respect to that specific subject.

Since sterilization is a medical procedure, the question is one of a person's ability to consent to medical treatment. Without a legally effective (or valid) consent, medical intervention constitutes a battery. The underlying moral and legal premise is that a person has a right to control his or her body and is to be protected from unwanted and offensive contact. A legally effective consent has the following elements: (1) It is voluntary; (2) information is provided about (a) the procedure and its possible consequences, and (b) alternative procedures and their possible consequences; and (3) the person is capable of comprehending the information.[13] These conditions are morally justified, since coercion or lack of information prevents assent from being a deliberate choice indicating a person's true desires or will.

[11] *Relf* v. *Weinberger*, 372 F. Supp. 1196, 1202 (D. D.C. 1974). See Appendix (p. 209) for text.

[12] G. S. Neuwirth; P. A. Hersler; & K. S. Goldrich, "Capacity, Competence, Consent: Voluntary Sterilization of the Mentally Retarded," *Columbia Human Rights Law Review* 6 (1975): 451.

[13] *Relf* v. *Weinberger*, 273 F. Supp. 1196, 1202 (D. D.C. 1974); *Cobbs* v. *Grant*, 8 Cal. 3d 229, 502 P. 2d 1, 104 Cal. Rptr. 505 (1972).

There are two main difficulties with consent to sterilization by the mentally incompetent. First, whereas some mentally incompetent persons may clearly have the specific capacity to comprehend the requisite information, others may not. The frequent irreversibility of sterilization may make it a more crucial decision than a contract or even marriage; and the ability to comprehend and assess such permanent effects requires considerable mental capacity. Second, the mentally incompetent, particularly the retarded, are especially vulnerable to suggestions of others; they have a strong desire for approval.[14] Moreover, the mentally incompetent have often been subject to various forms of coercion to consent.[15]

Committees

Because of possible coercion, proposals have been made for committees to review the consent of the mentally incompetent to sterilization, and one court has required it for all residents of an institution.[16] Various procedural elements are involved in these proposals, but the main ones are that a review committee be independent (no member being involved in the sterilization or employed at an institution in which the person is an inmate) and that a lawyer represent the person. The other elements are standard procedural ones of notice, right to cross-examine, and so on. Two crucial issues about such a procedure concern when it should be used and what precisely the committee is to determine.

Committee review involves a rather complicated procedure which might well deter even a mentally competent person from seeking sterilization. Moreover, the mentally incompetent would have more difficulty than the competent appropriately following all the procedures. If a review were

[14]R. Soskin, "Voluntary Sterilization: Safeguarding Freedom of Choice," *Amicus* (February 1977): 41.

[15]Neuwirth et al., "Capacity, Competence, Consent."

[16]Neuwirth et al., 464–69; *Wyatt* v. *Aderholt*, 368 F. Supp. 1383, 1385 (M.D. Ala. 1974).

required for sterilization of every mentally incompetent person, it would impose a significant impediment to the exercise of fundamental rights with respect to procreation. Moreover, a physician is and should be legally liable for performing a sterilization without a valid consent. In questionable cases, a physician may obtain a second opinion about the validity of a mental incompetent's consent. The fear of a malpractice suit should ensure that a physician would request a committee review, if it were available, in cases in which the validity of a person's consent remained questionable. Thus, making committee review available but not required is likely to provide adequate safeguard for consents to sterilization by mentally incompetent persons not institutionally confined.

However, committee review may be needed for all institutionalized incompetents. In their case, the voluntariness of the consent is more often questionable. A community physician has some assurance of voluntariness because the person comes to him, although undue influence or pressure may have been exerted by family or social workers. But in an institutional setting, many people may influence and pressure inmates to be sterilized. Moreover, there may be a tacit assumption that sterilization is a necessary condition for release. Finally, it is more convenient for patients and administratively easier to have a committee review of all cases in an institution than it is of all cases arising in community practice. These are good reasons to require committee review for all voluntary sterilizations of institutionalized incompetents.

INVOLUNTARY STERILIZATION

Sterilization of a person incapable of valid consent is involuntary and should only be permitted by a court order. The doctrine of "substituted consent" is sometimes used to classify sterilizations of the mentally incompetent as voluntary. By this doctrine, a parent or other legal guardian is permitted to consent to medical procedures for his child or ward. However, in these cases the person herself does not provide a valid consent; someone else consents in her behalf. Various commentators have noted that the interests of parents and mentally incompetent children may diverge.[17] Parents may fear that if their child begets offspring, they would ultimately have the primary burden of raising them. Moreover, sterilization of a mentally incompetent child may make her care easier, since there would be fewer problems concerning sexual activity or contraception. This divergence of interests may not arise with respect to court-appointed guardians, especially lawyers appointed as guardians. However, it is almost as easy for courts themselves to determine the appropriateness of sterilization as it is for them to ensure full legal protection of the rights of the mentally incompetent. Consequently, substituted consent should not be permitted.

There are two distinct groups of persons who might be subject to involuntary sterilization. As was just argued, all those persons incapable of valid consent to sterilization can only be sterilized involuntarily, or better, nonvoluntarily. The other group consists of persons who are capable of valid consent to sterilization but might be ordered sterilized without it.

There is one significant difference between the rationales that may justify sterilization of these two groups. Under its *parens patriae* power, the state is to protect the interests of a mental incompetent; and if sterilization would be in her best interest, a court may order it. Indeed, since the state is to act in the interests of the mentally incompetent, it fails to fulfill its responsibilities if a sterilization in the person's best interest is not performed. However, this rationale does not apply to those capable of valid consent. The paternalistic power of the state does not justifiably extend over these people in this respect. There are difficult questions as to what conditions

[17]Neuwirth et al., "Capacity, Competence, Consent," 455; Soskin, "Voluntary Sterilization," 42. Feminine pronouns are used to denote the mentally incompetent in this section since about two-thirds of involuntary sterilizations are performed on women.

indicate sterilization is in the best interest of a mental incompetent, and in the past this rationale has been too easily applied. Nonetheless, there are some cases in which sterilization is quite clearly in the person's best interest, just as there are for people who are competent. The reasons may, but need not, have anything to do with a person's incompetence.

OVERRIDING FUNDAMENTAL RIGHTS

The crucial question is whether there are any moral reasons which may justify involuntary sterilization of mental incompetents who are capable of valid consent. To do so, the reasons must override their fundamental rights with respect to procreation (to beget and rear children). Fundamental rights are legally protected by the due process clause of the Fourteenth Amendment to the Constitution; but they are not legally or morally absolute. Under the substantive due process doctrine, states may infringe fundamental rights only if there is a compelling state interest for so doing and the least restrictive alternative is used.[18]

Two general points should be noted about the least-restrictive-alternative requirement. First, unless a person is sexually active or is likely to be, no possible state concern with respect to her procreation arises. "Sexually active" means engaging in intercourse, not merely being sexually mature. Second, contraception must not be a feasible alternative. One possible alternative is compulsory injections of depo-provera, which provides three-month infertility in women. However, after depo-provera use it takes longer for fertility to return than with other forms of contraception, and it may have other side effects rendering it less desirable than surgical sterilization.

The basic issue is whether there are any compelling interests that would justify involuntary sterilization. There are general social interests—those of persons other than the in-

[18]See, for instance, *Roe* v. *Wade*, 410 U.S. 113 (1973); *Shelton* v. *Tucker*, 364 U.S. 479 (1960).

competent person and possible children. These interests primarily pertain to the general burdens that might be imposed upon society as a result of procreation by the mentally incompetent. If children might have genetic mental or physical defects or parents might require special supportive services, there will be additional burdens on society in providing care. However, since these burdens would primarily be financial, they do not by themselves justify sterilization.

However, as I noted in my opening paragraphs, courts have upheld statutes providing for involuntary sterilization on two general rationales: genetic well-being and parental incompetence. Thus the two interests that may be compelling are those concerning genetic well-being and parental nurture of children. Each of these interests provides a rationale for involuntary sterilization that requires closer examination.

THE GENETIC RATIONALE

Three key aspects of this rationale require consideration. The first concerns the seriousness of the likely defect: it must make a child incapable of attaining or taking advantage of minimum welfare or equality of opportunity. One approach would be to require the defect to be so serious that the child would be incompetent. However, this criterion only addresses possible mental defects. Although physical defects are not generally grounds for adjudging a person incompetent, the underlying reasoning might include both and a criterion should reflect that fact. A somewhat broader standard is that the child would be incapable of becoming an independent adult in the ordinary circumstances of life, including ramps for people confined to wheelchairs, and the like. Yet physical defects that would prevent children from obtaining a living—paralysis from the neck down—would probably be serious enough to justify involuntary sterilization. However, defects that would not prevent a person from earning a living and functioning in society would not be sufficiently serious.

The second aspect concerns how probable it is that a child born of mentally incompetent parents would be so handicapped. Every couple has some chance of begetting a defective child. For "normal" women over 35 years of age, the probability of having a child with Down's syndrome approaches 1 in 100. Since everyone has some chance of begetting a child with a genetic defect, it must be known that there is a genetic condition likely to produce such a child. Many mental illnesses and much mental retardation are not known to be genetically based. The difficult issue is how likely it must be that a child will have a defect. No absolute probability such as 25 percent can be specified as a minimum. Instead, the probability sufficient to justify sterilization will vary with the seriousness of the defect; the more serious it is, the smaller the probability needed to justify a sterilization.

The third aspect concerns possible less restrictive alternatives. For some genetic defects, amniocentesis and selective abortion of defective fetuses are possible. If a person is capable of being a competent parent, then selective abortion is a less restrictive alternative. Moreover, if the person suffers the defect and is still capable of being a competent parent, then the defect is probably not serious enough to justify sterilization. However, in rare cases it might be. Finally, if retarded males are capable of being parents but at risk for transmitting genetic defects, artificial insemination of their spouse by a donor preserves the right to rear children despite sterilization.

THE PARENTAL-INCOMPETENCE RATIONALE

This rationale concerns not only the right to beget children but also that to rear children. In the absence of a condition known to be genetic, merely requiring adoption of any children who are born may be a possible, less restrictive alternative. The children are capable of attaining and taking advantage of minimum welfare and equality of opportunity. Moreover, although the right to rear children would be denied, that to beget children would be preserved. However, there is no assurance that couples would be available immediately to adopt children, especially if they know a genetic parent was incompetent. Moreover, the rearing of infants in public institutions is often unsuccessful; many fail to thrive and die. Since incompetent persons would be denied the more valuable right to rear children, only the less valuable right to beget children would be relevant. When the social interest in avoiding burdens is added to the concern about the nurture of children, the two together are sufficiently compelling to prevail over the right to beget children.

The most difficult aspect of the parental-incompetence rationale is determining the incompetence. There are no clear sociological or psychological criteria for being a competent parent. However, there are two basic arguments pertaining to mental incompetence and capacity to be a competent parent. First, if a person is incapable of valid consent to sterilization, it is exceedingly doubtful that she is capable of being a competent parent. Such a person lacks a basic, specific capacity relevant to being a parent. A person who cannot comprehend the consequences of, and alternatives to, sterilization often lacks the basic capacity to understand long-range interests. A parent must consider and make judgments concerning a child's medical welfare. If a person is incapable of making such judgments for herself, then she is surely incapable of making them for others. Yet, the capacity validly to consent to sterilization does not demonstrate competence to be a parent. Competence to consent to sterilization pertains to a specific aspect of living and functioning, but the care of children requires many more and different capacities.

The second argument is more general and pertains to all the mentally incompetent. Simply stated, if a person cannot protect herself or manage her affairs, she is therefore incapable of being a competent parent. A parent is a legal guardian of her children, but one who requires a legal guardian herself is incapable of being a legal guardian of others. Although the nonlegal or factual criteria are disputable, one writer has remarked that parents with IQs less than 55 or 60 are seldom able to provide proper care of children.[19] Generally, the ca-

[19] J. E. Davis, "Birth Control by Sterilization," in Claude A. Frazier, ed., *Is It Moral to Modify Man?* (Springfield, Ill.: Charles C Thomas, 1973), pp. 75–76.

pacities for managing one's own affairs so overlap those of caring for children that it is doubtful that many persons lacking the former will nonetheless possess the latter.

A consideration weakens the force of these two arguments. Parental functions are usually shared by a couple. If one parent lacks the competence to perform certain parental tasks, the other parent may be capable of doing them. Consequently, in considering competence to be a parent, it is inappropriate to focus exclusively on the capacities of the mentally incompetent person, ignoring the possible competence of the partner. Nonetheless, given the high incidence of divorce and the possibility of premature death or incapacitation of the competent partner, it may be unwise to rest much faith upon the capacities of the mentally competent parent, at least without mandating that in the event of divorce or separation that parent receive custody of any children.

One final consideration: to justify involuntary sterilization, one must have evidence that the person's incompetent condition is probably permanent. The genetic rationale presents no problem on this point. However, it is important for the parental-incompetence rationale. Many mental illnesses are treatable and may not be permanent. Consequently, the parental-incompetence rationale applies to few people who are mentally incompetent because of mental illness. The situation with respect to mental retardation is less clear. With young children and adolescents, it is often not possible to predict their eventual level of functioning. Moreover, many residents of institutions, as many as 25 percent according to one author,[20] may be suffering correctable emotional or physical disabilities. It is not justifiable to sterilize the mentally retarded on the ground of parental incompetence until one

[20]W. Kempton, "Sexual Rights and Responsibilities of the Retarded Person," in *The Social Welfare Forum, 1976*, National Conference on Social Welfare (New York: Columbia University Press, 1977), pp. 217–218. An English court made an 11-year-old retarded girl a ward of the court to prevent her mother having her sterilized, because the court believed that by the time she was 18 the girl would be sufficiently competent to decide for herself; *Re D (a minor)* [1976] 1 A11 E.R. 326 (Fam. D.).

is reasonably sure there will not be sufficient improvement to render them competent parents. Hence, the parental-incompetence rationale does not justify involuntary sterilization of minor retarded persons (under age 18) when there is an alternative of involuntary contraception, such as IUDs or depo-provera injections for women.

CONCLUSION

Many mentally incompetent persons can validly consent to sterilization, and preventing their doing so infringes their rights with respect to procreation. However, appropriate safeguards are often needed to ensure the validity of their consent. Unless the person consents, sterilizations are involuntary and are justifiable only if ordered by a competent court after a hearing according due process of law.

There are three acceptable rationales for involuntary sterilizations, assuming that less restrictive alternatives are not feasible and that the person is, or is likely to be, sexually active. First, the person's best interest may justify sterilization of persons incapable of valid consent, but never of persons capable of valid consent. Second, involuntary sterilization of persons regardless of their capacity to validly consent is justifiable if there is a significant chance that their children would suffer a genetic defect preventing their development into adults capable of managing on their own in the ordinary circumstances of life. Third, involuntary sterilization of persons permanently incapable of being competent parents is justifiable; the inability validly to consent to sterilization is at least a strong indication that persons lack the competence to be parents, whereas general mental incompetence is a weaker indication.

CHAPTER 12

Sterilizing the Mildly Mentally Retarded without Their Consent

The Philosophical Arguments

ROBERT NEVILLE

Under certain specific circumstances it is morally permissible to sterilize some mildly mentally retarded people without their consent. At the outset of my argument I want to acknowledge that there is a grave difficulty, conceptually and empirically, in identifying which individuals belong to the relevant class of the mentally retarded. If that class is either

This Chapter was published soon after the completion of the project in the *Hastings Center Report* (June 1978).

ROBERT NEVILLE • Department of Philosophy and Center for Religious Studies, State University of New York at Stony Brook, Stony Brook, New York 11794.

conceptually so vague or empirically so confused that individuals who do not belong in it are inadvertently placed there, then it would be ethically impermissible to subject the class to involuntary sterilization. But let me put that difficulty aside until the end, and proceed with the argument as if we knew with acceptable exactness who the mildly mentally retarded are and which of them meet the specified requirements for sterilization.

THE HUMBLE ARGUMENT

My argument is really two arguments, one nested in the other. The first can be called the "humble argument" for involuntary sterilization, and it attempts to make the case that involuntary sterilization is in the best interest of certain mildly mentally retarded people. The second can be called the "philosophical argument," and it interprets the "humble argument" as a problem of rights and responsibilities, and attempts to show that involuntary sterilization in the right cases fosters rather than denies the membership of the mildly mentally retarded in the moral community.

The humble argument begins with certain observations. First, at least some mildly mentally retarded people are capable of engaging in and taking pleasure in heterosexual intercourse. My following remarks concern only this group; presumably those incapable of such intercourse would not need sterilization; those who, because of inexperience, do not know their capacities for pleasure should be viewed as capable of engaging in and taking pleasure from sexual activity until proved otherwise.

Second, for some mildly retarded people sexual activity is capable of being integrated into emotional aspects of affection, which can in turn contribute to positive, rewarding fulfillments of personal and social life. Freed from pregnancy, childbearing, and child rearing, an active heterosexual life can enrich the existence of some mildly mentally retarded people in much the way it can that of so-called "normals." Other things being equal, mildly mentally retarded people can benefit from and have a right to sexual activity and the social forms sexual relationships can involve, such as marriage. Capacities for marriage and long-lasting affection do not have to be clearly present, however, for the retarded to have a claim on sexual activity for purposes of pleasure alone.

Third, what begins to make the situation for the retarded "not equal" to that for "normals"? For mildly mentally retarded women the physiological and emotional changes that take place during pregnancy, and the violence of childbirth, are often experienced as disorienting and terrifying traumata. To the extent that a retarded man participates in the process, he too can be disoriented and lose his personal equilibrium.

Fourth, child rearing is sometimes beyond the capacities of mildly mentally retarded people precisely because of the characteristics of their retardation. The fact that child rearing is in practice also beyond the emotional capacities of many normal people should not obscure the overwhelming difficulty that it often poses for the retarded. Now it seems a prima facie argument that children ought not be conceived if there is not some reasonable expectation that they will receive minimal care. (Note that this is not an argument that conceived children should be aborted, which is more difficult to sustain.)

Fifth, mildly mentally retarded people have very great difficulty in managing impermanent forms of contraception. I am assuming that sterilization is the only permanent contraceptive; at least it cannot be reversed without medical help. Therefore, if these mildly mentally retarded people are to engage in sexual intercourse, which is otherwise desirable, without fear of the woman becoming pregnant, sterilization seems the only responsible contraceptive choice.

The humble argument, then, puts together these observations and says that the mildly mentally retarded people to whom these conditions apply should be sterilized so that they may enjoy heterosexual activity if they are so inclined. If they were not sterilized they would have to be prevented from engaging in sexual activity, or conditioned to homosexual or autoerotic sexual activity exclusively, which would be hard to guarantee. If their sex lives were not so controlled, they would run the risk of pregnancy with likely trauma for themselves and improper care for their child. If the retarded people do not or cannot give consent, then someone should have the standing to insist that the retarded be sterilized involuntarily.

An added consideration may be raised at the level of the humble argument. Who is to be sterilized, men, women, or both? The answer to that question clearly depends on the circumstances—whether the candidates are living in an institution, whether that institution is highly regulated or more informal in its management of personal associations; or, if the candidates are living outside institutions, in what kinds of settings. But generally the point of sterilization is to maximize the freedom of the mildly mentally retarded in sexual matters, and it is relevant to administer the procedure to any candidate meeting the conditions who stands to suffer harm or loss of freedom without it.

THE PHILOSOPHICAL ARGUMENT

The humble argument is a fairly straightforward, prudential argument operating within the limits and categories generally taken for granted when dealing with the mildly mentally retarded. The philosophical argument differs by calling into question the limits and categories otherwise taken for granted.

My philosophical argument consists of two main parts. The first considers the objection that sterilization of the mildly mentally retarded is wrong if done involuntarily because it would thereby deny the subjects their proper place in the moral community, treating them as means only and not ends in themselves. I shall argue on the contrary that the procedure enhances the dignity of their position in the moral community. The second part raises the very large problem of who decides about sterilization in the context of the mildly mentally retarded. Whereas some people might argue that no third party has sufficient standing in the matter to warrant doing violence to the candidate, I shall argue that it is the responsibility (a) of the moral community to establish policy creating such standing, and (b) of its properly delegated representatives to carry out the policy subject to a variety of checks.

MEMBERSHIP IN THE MORAL COMMUNITY

In that tradition of Western theory which takes most seriously the dignity of the human individual, the Kantian, one of the central concepts is that of the moral community. The dignity that should be accorded to each person as a human being consists in being regarded as a member of the moral community. Membership in that community means that a person is held to be morally responsible for his or her actions and life, and is to be held responsible by the rest of the community for assuming that responsibility.

With respect to human dignity, the grave danger is that a person will be treated as a thing rather than a responsible agent. This may happen when someone or some group treats a person merely as a means toward their own ends; this was Immanuel Kant's particular worry. It may also happen when the community simply fails to recognize the person as a moral agent, which happens most often when people's behavior is explained in such a way as to shift responsibility onto causes other than themselves. This objectification or alienation has been a primary worry of existentialists and many other social critics. In a strict philosophical sense (deriving from Aristotle), violence is done to people when they are prevented by external forces from fulfilling their basic or natural goals; one form of violence is to prevent someone from exercising membership in the moral community.

The mildly retarded suffer enough from their incapacities

that special care should be taken to ensure them as full a membership in the moral community as possible. To sterilize them involuntarily, some people argue, is to do them unnecessary and dehumanizing violence. It is to regard them first of all as incapable of making a responsible decision about sterilization, thus ruling them out of membership in this respect; no defender of involuntary sterilization could deny this fact. It is, second, to regard their sex lives and childbearing and child rearing lives as so controlled by irresponsible impulses that the people may just as well be managed like objects in those areas of life. Third, it is quite possible and indeed likely, according to this position, that sterilization is sought for the mildly mentally retarded in order to make their custody easier, in which cases the people are treated in that respect as means only, not as ends in themselves.

In answer to these arguments let me point out three characteristics of the moral community. First, membership in the moral community is relative to the capacity for taking moral responsibility; there is no membership in the moral community under ordinary circumstances in the respects in which there is no capacity for taking responsibility. Second, most capacities for taking moral responsibility need to be developed; ordinary socialization develops most of them. The state of moral adulthood can be defined as being in possession of the capacity to take responsibility for developing the other capacities for responsible action that might be called upon. Third, a general moral imperative for any community is that its structures and practices foster the development of the capacities for responsible behavior wherever possible, and avoid hindering that development.

The idea of a moral community is an ideal that exists in pure form only in the imagination. When the ideal is applied to actual communities, it must be tailored to the fact that some people can have only partial memberships because of limited capacity for morally responsible behavior. Children, for example, only slowly take on the capacities for full membership in the moral community, and come to be treated as full members by degrees. Ordinarily we think of young children as full human beings because of their potential to develop into adults with full capacity for responsible action; when the coherence of their lives is extended over a reasonable life span, they can be expected to have moral capacities in due season.

Other people have other sorts of limited capacities for responsible behavior, such as those resulting from mental illness or senility, in which certain areas of life may involve severe incapacities for responsible behavior whereas others do not. In these cases, we usually regard people as fully human members of the moral community by according them the rights of responsibility where they do in fact have the capacity and by assigning to other people the responsibilities of proxy in areas of incapacity. The concept of a proxy, in the restrictive use of my distinction, is that of an agent who fits into the patient's overall moral responsibility as a substitute in a certain area or under certain circumstances; the concept of proxy is used to maintain and support the notion that a person is a member of the moral community in circumstances where the direct capacity for that is lacking.

The case of the mildly mentally retarded is somewhat different from that of children and from the limited capacity of the mentally ill or senile. Like children, their capacities for development may be far greater than would have been imagined a few years ago. But unlike children, the pacing and sequencing of their development does not lead to emotional maturity at the same time they reach bodily maturity. For instance, the emotional and intellectual capacities to manage conventional birth control methods, to adjust to pregnancy, or to raise children do not develop by the time their physical development and their social peers among nonretarded people are ready for sexual activity.

Neither, sometimes, does the capacity to make informed decisions about sterilization. Indeed, if one were to say that heterosexual activity should be prevented among certain mildly mentally retarded people until such time as they develop the capacities for responsible behavior regarding pregnancy, or for consenting to surgical sterilization, the result is very likely to be the prevention of heterosexual activity altogether. As the humble argument says, this approach would amount to preventing the development of an important capacity for responsible behavior in areas that would be possible if an active sex life were possible, and would therefore be contrary to the imperative that the moral community foster such capacities.

Mildly mentally retarded people are like certain kinds of mentally ill people in that, from the adult perspective, there are certain areas of life in which they may lack capacities for responsible behavior and other areas where they may have them. But they are unlike mentally ill people in an important respect. A mentally ill person is conceived to be a member of the moral community because even though a proxy might exercise some of his or her responsibilities, he or she is believed to have the structure of a person who possesses the capacities for those responsibilities.

This belief is based on the fact, for instance, that the person once exercised those responsibilities before becoming ill. With the help of a proxy, almost as a prosthetic device, a mentally ill person can be presented to the moral community as a fully responsible moral agent. A mildly mentally retarded person, however, lacks the full personality structure that would come from having had the capacities for morally responsible behavior in the past. Although another person might make decisions in areas in which the retarded person is incapacitated, that would not strictly speaking be a case of proxy because the retarded person does not have a personality structured around the capacity for which a proxy might have to substitute.

Paternalism and proxy are models for enabling persons—children and the mentally ill, respectively—to enjoy membership in the moral community when they themselves have capacities for only partial membership. Another model is needed for the limited capacity of mildly mentally retarded people, one which I propose to call the model of "involuntary restrictive conditions." The model depicts mildly mentally retarded people as members of the moral community on the condition that they meet certain restrictions. Just as people with bad eyesight may be licensed to drive with the restriction that they wear glasses, so mildly mentally retarded people may be required to meet certain restrictions in order to be members of the moral community.

The analogy with driver's licenses is imperfect, however, because a person with bad eyesight can always choose not to drive and thereby not to need to wear glasses. But a person cannot choose to be in or out of the moral community; one is either in the position to be held responsible or one is not. Mildly mentally retarded people, and perhaps other groups, must meet the restrictions as conditions for being in the community. Therefore, from the standpoint of mildly mentally retarded people, the restrictive conditions are involuntary.

In a moment I shall urge that sterilization may be a proper involuntary restrictive condition for membership in the moral community for mildly mentally retarded people, subject to the limitations mentioned in connection with the humble argument. Before that, however, I want to address the question of who decides about involuntary restrictive conditions.

Who Should Decide?

Whether a certain restrictive condition does indeed foster the capacity for responsible moral behavior is an empirical question. The suggestion has been made that, with sterilization, mildly mentally retarded people will be able to engage in the kind of sex life that can develop their capacities for responsible behavior in various human relationships. Without sterilization they either would be prevented from having sex, and therefore would not develop those capacities for sexual affection and comradeship, or they would have sex and find themselves in such trouble that sexual affection and companionship would again be beyond them.

Furthermore, this empirical argument suggests that behavior having to do with sexual affection and companionship is more important than what mildly mentally retarded people might gain from opportunities for pregnancy, childbirth, and child rearing. The first "who decides" question is: Who decides whether that empirical argument is right? I suggest that this decision is a broad social one, which should be as informed as possible by experts in all the relevant fields, including both mental retardation and ethics. Clearly that argument will always be under redefinition and refinement.

But the next "who decides" question is: Who sets the policies regarding the treatment of the mildly mentally retarded? The answer is that the decision must come from the political process (again informed by relevant experts, and formulated by broad intellectual dialogue). The reason for locating the decision in the political process is that that is the only legitimate way by which individuals can be dealt with against their wills by due process. But there are two normative factors within the political process. One is that the process should conform to whatever political norm structures it—for instance, that of a representative democracy. According to this factor, what the political process decides about mildly mentally retarded people is legitimate if due political procedures have been followed. The other normative factor, however, is the demands of being a moral community, since the political process is the vehicle for actualizing those demands. A political decision is moral if it accords with what is required as a minimum for a moral community.

If the sterilization of mildly mentally retarded people, subject to appropriate limitations, does indeed foster important capacities for morally responsible behavior, and if a moral community ought to foster such capacities where possible, the warrant for politically deciding to sterilize certain mildly mentally retarded people is a moral one, not merely one of political legitimacy. There is a prima facie obligation to foster people's capacity for responsibility, since this capacity is the basis of their membership in the moral community. Paradoxically, to refrain from sterilization is to do them the violence of preventing them from participating in the moral community in one of the important respects of which they are capable.

Assuming that the political process results in a sterilization policy, by what procedures and what officers should decisions be made about particular candidates? That is a prudential political question that I shall not attempt to address. It is necessary at this point, however, to refer to what Hastings Center lore calls the "klutz factor," namely, that translating a theoretical moral argument into a public policy with significant effects is likely to lead to blunders and abuse. Because of the "klutz factor," prudence may very well dictate that policies should be far more conservative than morality otherwise would dictate.

For instance, as I stated the "humble argument," the candidates for involuntary sterilization should include those who are capable of engaging in and taking pleasure in heterosexual activity, and yet who are incapable of taking responsibility for this activity in regards to pregnancy and the rest. This is a positive argument for sterilizing a class of people. In light of the "klutz factor," according to which the wrong people might be sent to the surgeon, perhaps it would be a prudent extra restriction to insist that candidates have demonstrated their need for sterilization by having already gotten into trouble by their sexual activity. I am not sure how to prevent such a restriction from being turned into a punitive measure against the retarded, however.

In general, with regard to all the "who decides" questions, it is important to make sure that the process of decision is self-critical and that opposition to any point of view is always funded as a corrective support.

UNIFYING THE ARGUMENTS

The philosophical side of the argument has intended to show that, contrary to the beliefs of some, involuntary sterilization does not involve treating the mildly mentally retarded as if they were not members of the moral community;

rather, it acknowledges real incapacities and neutralizes their effects, thereby enabling other capacities to be realized. Furthermore, if sterilization does in some important ways lead to the development of greater capacities for responsibility, then it is part of the obligation a society owes to its potential members to provide it, subject to appropriate protections against abuse. If a mildly mentally retarded person lacks the capacity to give or withhold informed consent because he or she does not understand the subtle issues involved, then having the decision made by the society's agents is one of the involuntary restrictive conditions that might help place the person in the community. The society has the prima facie obligation to make that decision and should do so unless other considerations prevail.

The basic philosophical principle involved in this argument is that a moral community has the social responsibility to foster capacities for morally responsible behavior. It should do so paternalistically in the case of children; it should do so with appropriate proxies in the case of impaired capacities; and it should do so through the institution of involuntary restrictive conditions in the case of basic human capacities that are undevelopable only in a future that is too late for other valuable capacities to be developed that otherwise would have been possible.

This reasoning brings us back to the "humble argument." From a philosophical point of view, the humble argument might well be valid. At least it is not wrong by virtue of violating the canons of membership in the moral community; it does not deny human dignity. Indeed, the structure of the humble argument is to provide for the dignity of humane heterosexual relations by removing the unbearable complications of potential pregnancy. Whether its premises are valid is an empirical matter.

Let me close by dealing with the question of adequate diagnosis of the appropriate conditions for involuntary sterilization. Some structure must be worked out to determine appropriate subjects. We have seen that to do so requires two sorts of determinations. The first is whether informed and emotionally balanced decisions regarding sterilization are within the capacities of the candidates; if they are, then the candidates' word should be decisive, and if they prefer nonsterilization then society should respect that choice, whatever other compensatory restrictions it requires (such as no sexual activity). The second is whether the candidates are capable of heterosexual intercourse but not capable of coping adequately with pregnancy, childbirth, and child rearing. Not all mentally retarded people would fall into this category, and specific empirical criteria would have to be developed before a program of involuntary sterilization could be instituted.

If no mildly mentally retarded people can be found who fall into this category, then none of them should be involuntarily sterilized. The consequence of this requirement is that the validity of involuntary-sterilization programs depends upon the development of criteria and diagnostic skills sufficient to discriminate the proper category of people. There have been disagreements concerning whether the definitions of relevant characteristics, and diagnostic skills for discerning them, are sufficiently developed to provide a capacity for responsible programs. In the face of excessive modesty and caution it should be pointed out that people are now classified as mildly mentally retarded and subjected to programs intended to help them.

There is one final point. It is sometimes believed that there is a totalitarian impetus lurking in any social policy that might require people to be good—in this case, to submit to involuntary restrictive conditions in order to develop the amiable responsibilities of a decent sex life. I admit that there is a danger, but urge that it be guarded against by specific safeguards and internal critical mechanisms rather than by a blanket rejection. If people could be whole and fully responsible by themselves, society would have no positive responsibilities, only negative, peace-keeping ones. But because people become responsible through the grace of social life, and because some people need special help in exercising responsibility, society does have positive duties in developing the capacity for responsible moral behavior.

Bibliography

Accreditation Council for Services for Mentally Retarded and Other Developmentally Disabled Persons, *Standards for Services for Developmentally Disabled Individuals*. Chicago: Joint Commission on Accreditation of Hospitals, 1977, revised April, 1979.

Affleck, Glenn, "Role-taking Ability and Interpersonal Conflict Resolution among Retarded Young Adults." *American Journal of Mental Deficiency* 80 (1975): 233–236.

Affleck, Glenn, "Role-taking Ability and the Interpersonal Competencies of Retarded Children." *American Journal of Mental Deficiency* 80 (1975): 312–316.

Baumeister, A.A., "The American Residential Institution: Its History and Character." In: Baumeister, A.A. and Butterfield, E., eds., *Residential Facilities for the Mentally Retarded*. Chicago: Aldine, 1970.

Blatt, Burton and Kaplan, F., *Christmas in Purgatory: A Photographic Essay on Mental Retardation* (2nd ed.) Boston: Allyn & Bacon, 1966. (Also published in Syracuse, N.Y.: Human Policy Press, 1974 [3rd ed.].)

Blatt, Burton, *Exodus from Pandemonium: Human Abuse and a Reformation of Public Policy*. Boston: Allyn & Bacon, 1970.

Blatt, Burton, *Souls in Extremis: An Anthology on Victims and Victimizers*. Boston: Allyn & Bacon, 1973.

Blatt, Burton, *Revolt of the Idiots: A Story*. Glen Ridge, N.J.: Exceptional Press, 1976.

Blatt, Burton, Bikelen, D. and Bogdan, R., *An Alternative Textbook in Special Education: People, Schools and Other Institutions*. Denver: Love Publishing, 1977.

Blatt, Burton, Ozolins, A., and McNally, J., *The Family Papers: A Return to Purgatory*. New York: Longman, 1979.

Braginsky, Dorothea D. and Braginsky, Benjamin M., *Hansels and Gretels*. New York: Holt, Rinehart & Winston, 1971.

Burt, Robert A., "Beyond the Right to Habilitation." In: Kindred, M., Cohen, J., Penrod, D. and Shaffer, T., eds., *The Mentally Retarded Citizen and the Law*. New York: Free Press, 1976.

Cagelka, W.J. and Tyler, J.L., "Efficacy of Special Class Placement." *Training School Bulletin* 67 (1970): 33–68.

Cleary, T., Humphreys, L.G., Kendrick, S.A. and Wesman, A., "Educational Uses of Tests with Disadvantaged Students." *American Psychologist* 30 (1975): 15–41.

Conley, R., *The Economics of Mental Retardation*. Baltimore: Johns Hopkins University Press, 1973.

Conley, R., "Mental Retardation: An Economist's Approach." *Mental Retardation* 14 (1976): 6.

Edgerton, Robert, *The Cloak of Competence*. Berkeley: University of California Press, 1967.

The Fleischmann Report on the Quality, Cost, and Financing of Elementary and Secondary Education in New York State. New York: Viking Press, 1973.

Gan, J., Tymchuck, A.T. and Nishihara, A., "Mildly Retarded Adults: Their Attitudes toward Retardation." *Mental Retardation* 15 (1977): 5–9.

Goffman, E., *Asylums*. Chicago: Aldine, 1961.

Guidelines for the Use of Behavior Procedures in State Programs for Retarded Persons. A monograph series, 1 (1). Arlington Tex.: National Association for Retarded Citizens, Research Advisory Committee, 1975.

Hobbs, Nicholas, *The Future of Children*. San Francisco: Jossey-Bass, 1974.

Horrobin, J.M. and Rynders, J.E., *To Give an Edge*. Minneapolis: Colwell Press, 1972.

Inhelder, B. and Piaget, J., *The Growth of Logical Thinking from Childhood to Adolescence*. New York: Basic Books, 1958.

Itard, Jean Marc Gaspard, *The Wild Boy of Aveyron*. New York: The Century Company, 1932.

Kanner, L., *A History of the Care and Study of the Mentally Retarded*. Springfield, Ill.: Charles C Thomas, 1964.

Kershner, J.R., "Conservation of Vertical-Horizontal Space Perception in Trainable Retarded Children." *American Journal of Mental Deficiency* 77 (1973): 710–716.

Kramer, J.R., "The Right Not to Be Mentally Retarded." In: Kindred, M., Cohen, J., Penrod, D. and Shaffer, T. eds., *The Mentally Retarded Citizen and the Law*. New York: Free Press (1976).

Lemert, E.M., *Human Deviance, Social Problems and Social Control*. Englewood Cliffs, N.J.: Prentice-Hall, 1967.

Lippman, Leopold and Goldberg, I. Ignacy, *Right to Education: Anatomy of the Pennsylvania Case and Its Implications for Exceptional Children*. New York: Teachers College Press, 1973.

Lovell, K., "The Developmental Approach of Jean Piaget." In: Garrison, M., ed., "Cognitive Models and Development in Mental Retardation." *American Journal of Mental Deficiency* 70 (1966): 84–95. (Monograph supplement.)

McKinnon, J.W. and Renner, J.W., "Are Colleges Concerned with Intellectual Development?" *American Journal of Physics* 39 (1971): 1047–1052.

Menolascino, F.J., ed., *Psychiatric Approaches to Mental Retardation*. New York: Basic Books, 1971.

Mercer, J., *Labeling the Mentally Retarded: Clinical and Social Perspectives on Mental Retardation*. Berkeley: University of California Press, 1973.

Piaget, J., Preface to the first edition of B. Inhelder, *Diagnosis of Reasoning in the Mentally Retarded*. New York: John Day, 1968.

Piaget, J., "Intellectual Evolution from Adolescence to Adulthood." *Human Development* 15 (1972): 1–12.

Piaget, J. and Inhelder, B., *The Psychology of the Child*. New York: Basic Books, 1969.

Robinson, N.M. and Robinson, H.B., *The Mentally Retarded Child : A Psychological Approach*. New York: McGraw-Hill, 1976.

Roos, P., "Current Issues in Residential Care with Special Reference to the Problems of Institutional Care." *Symposium on Residential Care for the Mentally Retarded*. Frankfurt, Germany: September 14–18, 1969. Arlington, Tex.: National Association for Retarded Citizens, 1969.

Roos, P., "Trends and Issues in Special Education for the Mentally Retarded." *Education and Training of the Mentally Retarded* 5 (1970): 51–61.

Roos, P., "Parent organizations." In: Wortis, J., ed., *Mental Retardation : An Annual Review, II*. New York: Grune & Stratton, 1970.

Roos, P., "Evolutionary Changes of the Residential Facility." In: Baumeister, A.A. and Butterfield, E., eds., *Residential Facilities for the Mentally Retarded*. Chicago: Aldine, 1970.

Roos, P., "Human Rights and Behavior Modification." *Mental Retardation* 12 (1974): 3.

Roos, P., "Psychological Impact of Sterilization on the Individual." *Law and Psychology Review*, School of Law. Birmingham: University of Alabama, (Spring 1975): 44–56.

Roos, P., "Parents and Families of the Mentally Retarded." In: Kauffman, James and Payne, James S., eds., *Mental Retardation: Introduction and Personal Perspectives*. New York: Charles E. Merrill, 1975.

Roos, P., "Trends in Residential Institutions for the Mentally Retarded." In: *Trends in Education*. Columbus, Ohio: University Council for Educational Administration, 1976.

Roos, P., "Action Implications of the Developmental Model." *Symposium on Early Intervention: Steps in the Prevention of Developmental Handicaps*. Parsons, Kans.: Parsons State Hospital and Training Center (April 27, 1976).

Roos, P., "Human Rights and Behavior Modification." In: *Token Economies in Rehabilitation: A Book of Readings*. Wisconsin: Materials Development Center, University of Wisconsin, 1976.

Roos, P., "Parents of Mentally Retarded Persons." *International Journal of Mental Health* 6 (1977): 96–119.

Roos, P., "The Law and Mentally Retarded People: An Uncertain Future" *Stanford Law Review* 31; (4) (1979): 613–624.

Roos, P. and McCann, B., "Major Trends in Mental Retardation" *International Journal of Mental Health* 6 (1977): 3–20.

Sarason, Seymour B. and Doris, John, *Psychological Problems in Mental Deficiency* (4th ed.) New York: Harper & Brothers, 1969.

Sargen, M.S., "Labeling and Classification." In: Kindred, M., Cohen, J., Penrod, D. and Shaffer, T., eds. *The Mentally Retarded Citizen and the Law*. New York: Free Press, 1976.

Schwebel, M., "Formal Operations in First Year College Students," *Journal of Psychology* 91 (1975): 133–141.

Seagoe, M.V., *Yesterday Was Tuesday, All Day, All Night*. Boston: Little, Brown, 1964.

Suffer the Children: The Politics of Health in Massachusetts. Boston: Beacon Press, 1970.

Turnbull, Ann P. and Turnbull, H. Rutherford, eds., *Parents Speak Out : Views from the Other Side of the Two-Way Mirror*. New York: Charles E. Merrill, 1978.

United Nations General Assembly, *Declaration on the Rights of Mentally Retarded Persons*. 26th Session, A/RES/2856 (XXVI), 1972.

Wald, P.M., "Basic Personal and Civil Rights." In: Kindred, M., Cohen, J., Penrod, D. and Shaffer, T., eds. *The Mentally Retarded Citizen and the Law*. New York: Free Press, 1976.

Wilton, K. and Boersman, F.J., "Conservation Research with the Mentally Retarded." In: Ellis, N.R., ed. *International Review of Research in Mental Retardation* (Vol. 7). New York: Academic Press, 1974.

Wolfensberger, W., *Normalization: The Principle of Normalization in Human Services*. Toronto: National Institute on Mental Retardation, 1972.

Woodward, M., "The Application of Piaget's Theory to Research in Mental Deficiency." In: Ellis, N.R., ed., *Handbook of Mental Deficiency*. New York: McGraw-Hill, 1963.

Wright, Beatrice, *Physical Disability : A Psychological Approach*. New York: Harper & Brothers, 1960.

Zigler, E., "Research on Personality Structure in the Retardate." In: Ellis, N.R., ed., *International Review of Research in Mental Retardation* (Vol. 1). New York: Academic Press, 1966.

Zigler, E., "Mental Retardation: Current Issues and Approaches." In: Hoffman, L.W. and Hoffman, M.L., eds. *Review of Child Development Research* (Vol. 2). New York: Russell Sage Foundation, 1966.

Zigler, E., "Familial Mental Retardation: A Continuing Dilemma," *Science* 155 (1967): 292–298.

Zigler, E., "Developmental versus Difference Theories in Mental Retardation and the Problem of Motivation," *American Journal of Mental Deficiency* 73 (1969): 536–556.

Zigler, E., "The Retarded Child as a Whole Person." In: Routh, D.K., ed., *The Experimental Psychology of Mental Retardation*. Chicago: Aldine, 1973.

Appendix

Introduction

With one exception, the judicial opinions from which excerpts were selected for this Appendix are discussed in Parts I and II of the book. In order to give the reader a fuller picture of how the judicial reasoning proceeded in a number of key cases, we have chosen several cases that bring out different features of the debate about sterilizing the mentally retarded.

The landmark *Buck* v. *Bell* decision is discussed in Part I, Chapters 5 and 6, and also in Part II, Chapter 11. It is instructive to see how markedly the perceptions of both facts and values have changed in the half century since Justice Holmes rendered this opinion.

Decided in 1974, *Relf* v. *Weinberger* addresses a number of procedural and substantive questions concerning the competence of mentally retarded persons to grant consent for sterilizations. Although the opinion excerpted here focuses on the issue of federal funding for sterilizations, it also incorporates the detailed conditions that must be met in order to safeguard the rights of retarded persons. This case is discussed in Chapter 11.

The third opinion, also handed down in 1974, was the decision of a county court in the state of Wisconsin. Not mentioned in this book, the case is included in the Appendix because there were *no* previous cases dealing with this issue in Wisconsin, and it is useful to see how a court addresses the issue of sterilization of the retarded for the first time. The decision invokes the concept of the least restrictive alternative in denying the petition to consent to sterilization.

North Carolina Association for Retarded Children v. *State of North Carolina* is discussed at some length in Part I, Chapters 5 and 6. Judge Craven, the circuit judge in the case, remarked that this case "involves the whole panoply of constitutional rights of mentally retarded persons in North Carolina." The opinion addresses the nature of mental retardation, the question of whether sterilization of the retarded can ever be truly voluntary, who may be authorized to order sterilizations, and other topics central to the debate in this book. It is included here because of the wide range of relevant issues brought out in the court's opinion.

Also discussed in Part I, Chapters 5 and 6 is the final case excerpted here, *Stump* v. *Sparkman*. Decided in 1978, this case may be familiar to readers of this book who recall newspaper accounts of a few years ago. A major portion of the court's opinion discusses whether or not a circuit judge is properly authorized to approve a petition, brought by the parents, for a (retarded) minor's sterilization. The court of appeals reversed a lower court's decision in this case, holding the judge immune from damages liability even if his approval of the petition was in error. The case is interesting for its demonstration of the serpentine windings of case law, and the latter's ability to avoid confronting the central moral issues that come before the courts.

BUCK *v.* BELL, SUPERINTENDENT

ERROR TO THE SUPREME COURT OF APPEALS OF THE STATE OF VIRGINIA

No. 292. Argued April 22, 1927—Decided May 2, 1927

Mr. JUSTICE HOLMES delivered the opinion of the Court.

. . .The case comes here upon the contention that the statute authorizing the judgment is void under the Fourteenth Amendment as denying to the plaintiff in error due process of law and the equal protection of the laws.

Carrie Buck is a feeble minded white woman who was committed to the State Colony above mentioned in due form. She is the daughter of a feeble minded mother in the same institution, and the mother of an illegitimate feeble minded child. She was eighteen years old at the time of the trial of her case in the Circuit Court, Court, in the latter part of 1924. An Act of Virginia, approved March 20, 1924, recites that the health of the patient and the welfare of society may be promoted in certain cases by the sterilization of mental defectives, under careful safeguard, etc.; that the sterilization may be effected in males by vasectomy and in females by salpingectomy, without serious pain or substantial danger to life; that the Commonwealth is supporting in various institutions many defective persons who if now discharged would become a menace but if incapable of procreating might be discharged with safety and become self-supporting with benefit to themselves and to society; and that experience has shown that heredity plays an important part in the transmission of insanity, imbecility, etc. The statute then enacts that whenever the superintendent of certain institutions including the above named State Colony shall be of opinion that it is for the best interests of the patients and of society that an inmate under his care should be sexually sterilized, he may have the operation performed upon any patient afflicted with hereditary forms of insanity, imbecility, etc., on complying with the very careful provisions by which the act protects the patients from possible abuse.

The superintendent first presents a petition to the special board of directors of his hospital or colony, stating the facts and the grounds for his opinion, verified by affidavit. Notice of the petition and of the time and place of the hearing in the institution is to be served upon the inmate, and also upon his guardian, and if there is no guardian the superintendent is to apply to the Circuit Court of the County to appoint one. If the inmate is a minor notice also is to be given to his parents if any with a copy of the petition. The board is to see to it that the inmate may attend the hearings if desired by him or his guardian. The evidence is all to be reduced to writing, and after the board has made its order for or against the operation, the superintendent, or the inmate, or his guardian, may appeal to the Circuit Court of the County. The Circuit Court may consider the record of the board and the evidence before it and such other admissible evidence as may be offered, and may affirm, revise, or reverse the order of the board and enter such order as it deems just. Finally any party may apply to the Supreme Court of Appeals, which, if it grants the appeal, is to hear the case upon the record of the trial in the Circuit Court and may enter such order as it thinks the Circuit Court should have entered. There can be no doubt that so far as procedure is concerned the rights of the patient are most carefully considered, and as every step in this case was taken in scrupulous compliance with the statute and after months of observation, there is no doubt that in that respect the plaintiff in error has had due process of law.

The attack is not upon the procedure but upon the substantive law. It seems to be contended that in no circumstances could such an order be justified. It certainly is contended that the order cannot be justified upon the existing grounds. The judgment finds the facts that have been recited and that Carrie Buck "is the probable potential parent of socially inadequate offspring, likewise afflicted, that she may be sexually sterilized without detriment to her general health and that her welfare and that of society will be promoted by her sterilization," and thereupon makes the order. In view of the general declarations of the legislature and the specific findings of the Court, obviously we cannot say as matter of law that the grounds do not exist, and if they exist they justify the result. We have seen more than once that the public welfare may call upon the best citizens for their lives. It would be strange if it could not call upon those who already sap the strength of the State for these lesser sacrifices, often not felt to be such by those concerned, in order to prevent our being swamped with incompetence. It is better for all the world, if instead of waiting to execute degenerate offspring for crime, or to let them starve for their imbecility, society can prevent those who are manifestly unfit from continuing their kind. The principle that sustains compulsory vaccination is broad enough to cover cutting the Fallopian tubes. *Jacobson* v. *Massachusetts*, 197 U.S. 11. Three generations of imbeciles are enough.

But, it is said, however it might be if this reasoning were applied generally, it fails when it is confined to the small number who are in the institutions named and is not applied to the multitudes outside. It is the usual last resort of constitutional argument to point out shortcomings of this sort. But the answer is that the law does all that is needed when it does all that it can, indicates a policy, applies it to all within the lines, and seeks to bring within the lines all similarly situated so far and so fast as its means allow. Of course so far as the operations enable those who otherwise must be kept confined to be returned to the world, and thus open the asylum to others, the equality aimed at will be more nearly reached.

Judgment affirmed.

KATIE RELF ET AL., PLAINTIFFS
v. CASPAR W. WEINBERGER ET AL., DEFENDANTS

NATIONAL WELFARE RIGHTS ORGANIZATION, PLAINTIFF
v. CASPAR W. WEINBERGER ET AL., DEFENDANTS

UNITED STATES DISTRICT COURT
FOR THE DISTRICT OF COLUMBIA
MARCH 15, 1974

MEMORANDUM OPINION

GESELL, District Judge.

These two related cases, which have been consolidated with the consent of all parties, challenge the statutory authorization and constitutionality of regulations of the Department of Health, Education and Welfare (HEW) governing human sterilizations under programs and projects funded by the Department's Public Health Service and its Social and Rehabilitation Service. . . .

Congress has authorized the funding of a full range of family planning services under two basic procedures. The Public Health Service administers federal grants to state health agencies and to public and private projects for the provision of family planning services to the poor.

Although there is no specific reference to sterilization in any of the family planning statutes nor in the legislative history surrounding their passage, the Secretary has considered sterilization to fall within the general statutory scheme and Congress has been made aware of this position. But until recently, there were no particular rules or regulations governing the circumstances under which sterilizations could be funded under these statutes.

Sterilization of females or males is irreversible. The total number of these sterilizations is clearly of national significance. Few realize that over 16 percent of the married couples in this country between the ages of 20 and 39 have had a sterilization operation. Over the last few years, an estimated 100,000 to 150,000 low-income persons have been sterilized annually under federally funded programs. Virtually all of these people have been adults: only about 2,000 to 3,000 per year have been under 21 years of age and fewer than 300 have been under 18. There are no statistics in the record indicating what percentage of these patients were mentally incompetent.

Although Congress has been insistent that all family planning programs function on a purely voluntary basis, there is uncontroverted evidence in the record that minors and other incompetents have been sterilized with federal funds and that an indefinite number of poor people have been improperly coerced into accepting a sterilization operation under the threat that various federally supported welfare benefits would be withdrawn unless they submitted to irreversible sterilization. Patients receiving Medicaid assistance at childbirth are evidently the most frequent targets of this pressure, as the experiences of plaintiffs Waters and Walker illustrate. Mrs. Waters was actually refused medical assistance by her attending physician unless she submitted to a tubal ligation after the birth. Other examples were documented.

When such deplorable incidents began to receive nationwide public attention due to the experience of the Relf sisters in Alabama, the Secretary took steps to restrict the circumstances under which recipients of federal family planning funds could conduct sterilization operations. On August 3, 1973, the Department published in the Federal Register a notice of Guidelines for Sterilization Procedures under HEW Supported Programs. The notice directed that the policies set forth in the guidelines be implemented through regulations to be issued by the departmental agencies administering programs which provide federal financial assistance for family planning services. Notices of proposed rule making were duly published in the Federal Register on September 21, 1973. Interested persons were given an opportunity to participate in the rule making by submitting comments on the proposed regulations. Approximately 300 comments, including those of plaintiff NWRO, were received and reviewed by the Department. The final regulations here under attack were issued on February 6, 1974.

These regulations provide that projects and programs receiving PHS or SRS funds, whether for family planning or purely medical services, shall neither perform nor arrange for the performance of a nontherapeutic sterilization unless certain procedures are carried out. These vary depending upon whether the patient is, under state law, a legally competent adult, a legally competent person under the age of 18, a legally incompetent minor, or a mental incompetent. Briefly, they are as follows:

(1) Legally competent adults must give their "informed consent" to sterilization. Such consent must be evidenced by a written and signed document indicating, *inter alia,* that the patient is aware of the benefits and costs of sterilization and of the fact that he may withdraw from the operation without losing federal benefits.

(2) Legally competent persons under the age of 18 must also give such written consent. In these situations, a special Review Committee of independent persons from the community must also have determined that the proposed sterilization is in the best interest of the patient, taking into consideration (a) the expected mental and physical impact of pregnancy and motherhood on the patient, if female, or the

expected impact of fatherhood, if male, and (b) the expected immediate and long-term mental and physical impact of sterilization on the patient. The Review Committee must also (a) review appropriate medical, social and psychological information concerning the patient, including the age of the patient, alternative family planning methods, and the adequacy of consent, and (b) interview the patient, both parents of the patient (if available), and such other persons as in its judgment will contribute pertinent information. However, parental consent is not required.

(3) Legally incompetent minors must be afforded the above safeguards, and, in addition, a state court of competent jurisdiction must determine that the proposed sterilization is in the best interest of the patient.

(4) The sterilization of mental incompetents of all ages must also be sanctioned by a Review Committee and a court. However, personal consent is not required—it is enough that the patient's "representative" requests sterilization. Although defendants interpret the term "representative" to mean a person empowered under state law to consent to the sterilization on behalf of the patient, no such definition appears in the regulations themselves.

Plaintiffs do not oppose the voluntary sterilization of poor persons under federally funded programs. However, they contend that these regulations are both illegal and arbitrary because they authorize *involuntary* sterilizations, without statutory or constitutional justification. They argue forcefully that sterilization of minors or mental incompetents is necessarily involuntary in the nature of things. Further, they claim that sterilization of competent adults under these regulations can be undertaken without insuring that the request for sterilization is in actuality voluntary. The Secretary defends the regulations and insists that only "voluntary" sterilization is permitted under their terms. . . .

For the reasons developed below, the Court finds that the Secretary has no statutory authority under the family planning sections of the Social Security or Public Health Services Acts to fund the sterilization of any person incompetent under state law to consent to such an operation, whether because of minority or of mental deficiency. It also finds that the challenged regulations are arbitrary and unreasonable in that they fail to implement the congressional command that federal family planning funds not be used to coerce indigent patients into submitting to sterilization. In short, federally assisted family planning sterilizations are permissible only with the voluntary, knowing and uncoerced consent of individuals competent to give such consent. This result requires an injunction against substantial portions of the proposed regulations and their revision to insure that all sterilizations funded under the family planning sections are voluntary in the full sense of that term and that sterilization of incompetent minors and adults is prevented.

The dispute with regard to minors and mental incompetents centers around two aspects of the statutory language. On the one hand, Congress included in every section mentioning family planning a requirement that such services be voluntarily requested. On the other hand, these sections purport to offer family planning services to all poor people and two of them specifically include minors. The Secretary argues that this juxtaposition indicates that Congress intended that minors personally and incompetents through their representatives would be able to consent to sterilization under these sections. That conclusion is unwarranted.

Although the term "voluntary" is nowhere defined in the statutes under consideration, it is frequently encountered in the law. Even its dictionary definition assumes an exercise of free will and clearly precludes the existence of coercion or force. *Webster's Second New International Dictionary* 2858 (2d ed. 1961). And its use in the statutory and decisional law, at least when important human rights are at stake, entails a requirement that the individual have at his disposal the information necessary to make his decision and the mental competence to appreciate the significance of that information.

No person who is mentally incompetent can meet these standards, nor can the consent of a representative, however sufficient under state law, impute voluntariness to the individual actually undergoing irreversible sterilization. Minors would also appear to lack the knowledge, maturity and judgment to satisfy these standards with regard to such an important issue, whatever may be their competence to rely on devices or medication that temporarily frustrates procreation. This is the reasoning that provides the basis for the nearly universal common law and statutory rule that minors and mental incompetents cannot consent to medical operations.

The statutory references to minors and mental incompetents do not contradict this conclusion, for they appear only in the context of family planning services in general. Minors, for example, are not legally incompetent for all purposes, and many girls of child-bearing age are undoubtedly sufficiently aware of the relevant considerations to use temporary contraceptives that intrude far less on fundamental rights. However, the Secretary has not demonstrated and the Court cannot find that Congress deemed such children capable of voluntarily consenting to an irreversible operation involving the basic human right to procreate. Nor can the Court find, in the face of repeated warnings concerning voluntariness, that Congress authorized the imposition of such a serious deprivation upon mental incompetents at the will of an unspecified "representative."

The regulations also fail to provide the procedural safeguards necessary to insure that even competent adults voluntarily request sterilization. Plaintiffs would require an elaborate hearing process prior to the operation to remedy this problem. The Secretary, however, has determined that the consent document procedure set forth in the existing regulations is adequate in most instances to insure a knowledgeable decision, and the Court finds that this determination is not unreasonable. In one respect, however, the consent procedure must be improved. Even a fully informed individual cannot make a "voluntary" decision concerning sterilization if he has been subjected to coercion from doctors or project officers. . . .The present statutes were passed to facilitate only voluntary family planning and thus to assist the individual in the exercise of his voluntary right to govern his own procreation. Involuntary sterilization is not only distinguishable from these services, but diametrically so. It invades rather than compliments the right to procreate.

This controversy has arisen during a period of rapid change in the field of birth control. In recent years, through the efforts of dedicated proponents of family planning, birth control information and services have become widely available. Aided by the growing acceptance of family planning, medical science has steadily improved and diversified the techniques of birth prevention and control. Advancements in artificial insemination and in the understanding of genetic attributes are also affecting the decision to bear children. There are even suggestions in the scientific literature that the sex of children may soon be subject to parental control. And over this entire area lies the specter of overpopulation, with its possible impact upon the food supply, interpersonal relations, privacy, and the enjoyment of our "inalienable rights."

Surely the Federal Government must move cautiously in this area, under well-defined policies determined by Congress after full consideration of constitutional and far-reaching social implications. The dividing line between family planning and eugenics is murky. And yet the Secretary, through the regulations at issue, seeks to sanction one of the most drastic methods of population control—the involuntary, irreversible sterilization of men and women—without any legislative guidance. Whatever might be the merits of limiting irresponsible reproduction, which each year places increasing numbers of unwanted or mentally defective children into tax-supported institutions, it is for Congress and not individual social workers and physicians to determine the manner in which federal funds should be used to support such a program. We should not drift into a policy which has unfathomed implications and which permanently deprives unwilling or immature citizens of their ability to procreate without adequate legal safeguards and a legislative determination of the appropriate standards in light of the general welfare and of individual rights.

STATE OF WISCONSIN **IN PROBATE**

DANE COUNTY COURT BRANCH I

In the Matter of the Temporary Guardianship of MARY LOUISE ANDERSON	ORDER 5-67-1648

Hearing: August 15, 1974 and September 16, 1974

Before: Judge P. Charles Jones

Appearances: Temporary guardian, Mr. Rueben J. Anderson, in person, and by ATTORNEY EDWARD H. RIKKERS;

Ward, in person, and by her guardian *ad litem*, ATTORNEY KENT I. CARNELL;

FACTS

Mary Louise Anderson is a nineteen (19) year-old mentally retarded girl with an I.Q. of approximately 70 who is also subject to petit and grand mal epileptic seizures. Her father was appointed temporary guardian of her person and her estate on June 19, 1974.

On August 7, 1974 the temporary guardian petitioned for

an order authorizing him, as guardian, to consent to surgery to sterilize his daughter. Two hearings were held in the matter and the Court took the issue under advisement.

At the first hearing the guardian ad litem could not appear. The Court did receive testimony from both parents and the ward. All three favored the surgery. Filed with the Court were certifications from Dr. Thomas V. Geppert, Dr. Gamber F. Tegtmeyer and Ronald M. Sindberg, Ph.D., all in support of the surgery. Filed, also, was a consent to sterilization signed by the ward. At the completion of the hearing the Court continued the matter pending the guardian ad litem's report.

The guardian ad litem reviewed the transcript and requested further testimony. At the September 16, 1974 hearing additional testimony was taken from the ward's parents and from Dr. Robert Cooke, Vice Chancellor of the University of Wisconsin.

Following the hearing the guardian ad litem made an oral report in opposition to the petition for sterilization.

DECISION

There are no Wisconsin cases dealing with this sensitive question. No standards have been developed to apply to the question in Wisconsin. See, for example, standards laid down by the Federal District Court for the Middle District of Alabama, *Wyatt* v. *Aderholt* (1974), 368 F. Supp. 1383. The Court believes that the question is of such importance that standards must be developed to apply to this case and others.

Sterilization as used in this decision means "any medical or surgical operation or procedure which results in a patient's permanent inability to reproduce," *Id.* at 1384. Sterilization, therefore, is the most drastic form of birth control. It does not include temporary measures for birth control or contraception.

Authority to sterilize mentally retarded or other developmentally disabled persons must fall under the aegis of Ch. 880, *Wis. Stats.* as modified by Ch. 284, Laws of 1973. The person to be sterilized must be incompetent and in need of a guardian. A guardian of the person, once appointed by the Court, assumes the "care, custody and control" of the ward; Sec. 880.01 (1) *Wis. Stats.*

The primary function of a guardian of the person is to "provide for the care, comfort and maintenance of the ward," *Guardianship of Bose* (1967), 39 Wis. 2d 80, 87. Sterilization, because of its irreversibility, is too drastic a procedure to justify absent a specific court order. Regardless of the medical necessity that might be involved or what the guardian may perceive as the best interests of his ward, authorization to sterilize should only come from the Court after a full evidentiary hearing.

Therefore, the temporary guardian in this case was totally correct in petitioning the Court for a hearing to consider an order authorizing him to consent on behalf of his ward.

* * *

Recent cases in the related field of involuntary commitment of mentally ill persons have required the use of the concept of "less drastic alternatives," *Lake* v. *Cameron* (1966), 364 F 2d 657; *Lessard* v. *Schmidt* (1972), 349 F 2d 1078.

> Even though the governmental purpose be legitimate and substantial, that purpose cannot be pursued by means that broadly stifle fundamental personal liberties when the end can be more narrowly achieved. The breadth of legislative abridgment must be viewed in the light of less drastic means for achieving the same basic purpose." *Shelton* v. *Tucker* (1960), 364 US 479, 488.

This concept has now been incorporated into the Wisconsin guardianship statutes through Ch. 284, Laws of 1973. Sec 55.001 *Wis. Stats.* states the policy. In part it provides that protective services are

> to place the least possible restriction on personal liberty and exercise of constitutional rights consistent with due process and protection from abuse, exploitation and neglect.

Sterilization as a means to prevent unwanted pregnancy of a retarded woman must be considered a "protective service" under Ch. 284. As such, the Court must be satisfied that the evidence demonstrates the following findings:

1. That the procedure is a medical necessity or that the procedure is in the best interests of the ward; and

2. That all available less drastic alternatives have been investigated; and

3. That all available less drastic alternatives are unsuitable.

In light of these factors the petition before the Court must be denied. The evidence does not indicate that the surgical procedure is a medical necessity. Although there is some evidence that the procedure might be in the best interest of the ward, the guardian ad litem disagreed. It is the opinion of the Court that "any doubts as to such matters shall be resolved against proceeding with sterilization," *Wyatt* v. *Aderholt*, supra at 1385.

Finally, the testimony indicates that there are less drastic alternatives available that should be investigated by the temporary guardian. Either the use of birth control pills or the use of an inter-uterine device must be tried before this procedure can be authorized.

THEREFORE IT IS ORDERED that the petition to consent to sterilization is denied.

Dated: November / , 1974

By the Court:

P. Charles Jones, Judge
Dane County Court
Branch 1

NORTH CAROLINA ASSOCIATION FOR RETARDED CHILDREN ET AL., PLAINTIFFS

AND

UNITED STATES OF AMERICA, PLAINTIFF-INTERVENOR

v.

STATE OF NORTH CAROLINA ET AL., DEFENDANTS

Civ. No. 3050

UNITED STATES DISTRICT COURT FOR THE MIDDLE DISTRICT OF NORTH CAROLINA, RALEIGH DIVISION

OCTOBER 1, 1976

CRAVEN, Circuit Judge:

What is now before this three-judge court is a piece of a much more ambitious lawsuit that involves the whole panoply of constitutional rights of mentally retarded persons in North Carolina. Because the legislature of North Carolina has changed or repealed most of the statutes relating to the treatment, training, and education of retarded children, we have concluded that all such questions presented by the pleadings should be severed from the issue relating to the constitutionality of the sterilization statute as applied to mentally retarded persons. We have retained only the latter, and have remanded all other questions to a single judge of the Eastern District of North Carolina for decision.

I

Based upon the pleadings and documents received in evidence or judicially noticed, and upon the depositions and the live testimony heard at Wilmington, North Carolina, we make the following ultimate findings of fact:

1. The statute under attack is N.C. Gen. Stat. § § 35-36 through -50, entitled Article 7, Sterilization of Persons Mentally Ill and Mentally Retarded. Plaintiffs attack its constitutionality as applied and applicable to mentally retarded persons.

2. As defined by the American Association of Mental Deficiency, mental retardation refers to significantly subaverage general intellectual functioning existing concurrently with defects in adaptive behavior and manifested during the developmental period.

3. Another section of the same North Carolina Chapter defines mental defective as follows:

> A "mental defective" shall mean a person who is not mentally ill but whose mental development is so retarded that he has not acquired enough self-control, judgment, and discretion to manage himself and his affairs, and for whose own welfare or that of others, supervision, guidance, care, or control is necessary or advisable. The term shall be construed to include "feeble-minded," "idiot," and "imbecile."
>
> —N.C.Gen. Stat. § 35-1.1.

4. Sterilization is a drastic procedure, almost impossible to reverse in females and difficult and uncertain to reverse in males, that is intended to be permanent and prevent procreation. It is not, medically speaking, a dangerous procedure.

5. Most competent geneticists now reject Social Darwinism and doubt the premise implicit in Mr. Justice Holmes' incantation that ". . . three generations of imbeciles is enough." But however doubtful is the efficacy of sterilization to improve the quality of the human race, there is substantial medical opinion that it may be occasionally desirable and indicated. Not even Dr. Clements, who testified for the

United States and expressed strongly his general disapproval of sterilization of the mentally retarded, would go so far as to say that in an extreme case he would not use an involuntary sterilization statue if available. We think it a fair statement, from the expert testimony we have heard and read, to say that the best opinion presently is that rarely would a competent doctor recommend involuntary sterilization—but that he might do so in an extreme case. As a corollary to that proposition, it is also fair to say, we think, that prevalent medical opinion views with distaste even voluntary sterilization for the mentally retarded and is inclined to sanction it only as a last resort and in relatively extreme cases. In short, the medical and genetical experts are no longer sold on sterilization to benefit either retarded patients or the future of the Republic.

6. The statute under attack became effective January 1, 1975. Since that time, only one resident of a North Carolina mental retardation center had undergone sterilization pursuant to the statutory procedure.

7. Between June 1970 and April 1974, 23 sterilizations were performed upon residents of North Carolina's mental retardation centers pursuant to the provision of the preceding statute. Viewed over a longer time span, there has been a diminishing frequency in use of the sterilization procedure, reflecting, we think, diminishing confidence of medical doctors in its efficacy for any purpose except to prevent conception. That it will do.

8. Mental retardation is a difficult, complex phenomenon. The nature of retardation, its causes and effects are not susceptible to facile generalizations. The problem in this litigation is compounded in that the plaintiff class is very broadly defined, and included all mentally retarded persons in North Carolina, regardless of their ages, the causes of their retardation, the degree of their intellectual, mental and social capabilities, their prospects for future growth and development.

9. Some general propositions nevertheless must be regarded as established by the evidence in this case. We emphasize that the following statements do *not* apply to all or even a majority of the plaintiff class. All, however, are true with respect to at least some members of the class:

(a) Mental retardation in some cases has as its cause an identifiable genetic defect. Under some circumstances it is within the capability of modern medical and genetical science to establish that the genetic defect is inheritable and that there is a significant probability or substantial likelihood that the offspring of a mentally defective parent would also be retarded.

(b) Mental retardation in some cases can be traced to an environment which blocks or shrinks the mental and intellectual development of a child. Under some circumstances it is within the capability of modern medical and sociological science to determine that a mentally retarded parent or parents would be incapable of providing offspring with an environment in which a child could reasonably be expected to develop in a normal manner. As a corollary to this proposition, it is in some cases possible to predict with substantial accuracy that a mentally retarded person would be incapable of discharging the responsibilities of parenthood.

(c) While mentally retarded persons may be entitled to express themselves sexually, it can in some cases be determined that a mentally defective person does not understand or cannot appreciate the natural consequences of sexual activity. It can, likewise, be determined in some cases that the conception of a child is neither the intention nor the expectation of the sexually active mental retardate.

(d) Some mentally retarded persons who are sexually active may not want children. While many sexually active retarded persons are capable of employing various methods of birth control effectively, some are incapable of effective voluntary contraception.

(e) In rare and unusual cases, it can be medically determined that involuntary sterilization is in the best interests of either the mentally retarded person or the State or both.

II

The statute is applicable to persons "mentally ill" or "mentally retarded," but we are here concerned only with those provisions which relate to mentally retarded persons.

The statute authorizes both voluntary and involuntary sterilizations. It applies to mentally defective persons housed in state institutions and those who are not patients in state institutions. In the case of a patient who is confined in a state institution, the person in charge of the sterilization procedure is the director of the institution. For retarded persons not in state institutions, the key official is the county director of Social Services. The appropriate state or county official is authorized by the statute to petition the state district court for the sterilization of the mentally retarded person when it "may be considered in the best interest of the mental, moral, or physical improvement" of the retarded person, "or for the public good." The sterilization operation, whether voluntary or involuntary, is paid for by the State or the county in which the retarded person lives.

The statute expressly provides that sterilization operations shall only be performed by qualified, licensed North Carolina physicians and then only pursuant to an order issued by an appropriate state court. If the person to be sterilized wishes to select his own physician, he may do so but must then pay for the costs and expenses of the operation. Otherwise the physician is selected by the "petitioner," i.e., the director of the institution or the county director of Social Services.

Section 35-39 makes it the *duty* of the petitioner to institute sterilization proceedings under the following circumstances:

(1) when he feels that sterilization is in the best interests of the mental, moral, or physical improvement of the retarded person,

(2) when he feels that sterilization is in the best interests of the public at large,

(3) when, in his opinion, the retarded person "would be likely, unless sterilized, to procreate a child or children who would have a tendency to serious physical, mental, or nervous disease or deficiency; or, because of physical, mental, or nervous disease or deficiency which is not likely to materially improve, the person would be unable to care for a child or children."

(4) when the next of kin or legal guardian of the retarded person requests that he file the petition.

[1] We conclude that subparagraph 4 of Section 39 is irrational and irreconcilable with the first three subparagraphs. The first three paragraphs make out a complete and sensible scheme: that the public servant concern himself *either* with the best interest of the retarded person *or* the best interest of the public, or both, *and* that he act to begin the procedure *only* when in his opinion the retarded person would either likely procreate a defective child or would himself be unable to care for his own child or children. All of this makes sense. The fourth subparagraph does not. Instead, it grants to the retarded person's next of kin or legal guardian the power of a tyrant: for any reason, or for no reason at all, he may *require* an otherwise responsible public servant to initiate the procedure. This he may do without reference to any standard and without regard to the public interest or the interest of the retarded person. We think such confidence in *all* next of kin and *all* legal guardians is misplaced, and that the unstated premises of competency to decide to force initiation of the proceeding and never failing fidelity to the interest of the retarded person are invalid. We hold this subsection four unconstitutional as an arbitrary and capricious delegation of unbridled power and a correspondingly irrational withdrawal

of responsibility sensibly placed upon the director of the institution or the county director of Social Services by the other three coherent and compatible subparagraphs.

Written into § 35-39 are two fundamental but unarticulated premises. First, the statute presumes that it is possible in some cases to determine that the retarded person has a genetic defect which likely would be inherited by his children. Secondly, the statute presumes that some persons may be so severely retarded that they would be unable to properly care for a child should they conceive one. As determined in the findings of fact, *supra,* we are of the opinion that in some cases, rare though they may be, these two general presumptions inherent in the statute are valid.

The petition which is filed with the district court is required to contain information from which the district court will be able to make appropriate findings of fact and conclusions of law regarding the propriety of the requested sterilization operation. The petition must contain the results of psychological or psychiatric testing which support the petitioner's assertion that the retarded person is subject to the statute and must contain any statement by an examining physician which indicates "any known contra indication to the requested surgical procedure." The petition also requires the written consent or objection of the legal guardian or next of kin of the retarded person, and if there is none provides for appointment of a guardian ad litem "who *shall* make investigation and report to the court . . ." The petition "should also contain the consent or objection of the person upon whom the sterilization operation is to be performed." If the mentally retarded person is incapable of giving his consent or registering his objection, the petitioner must certify to the court that the procedure has been explained to the person.

A copy of the petition filed with the district court must be served upon the retarded person and his legal or natural guardian or a guardian ad litem or next of kin at least 20 days prior to the hearing on the petition. The district court is also authorized to conduct an investigation in certain circumstances.

After the petition is filed and upon appropriate notice to the retarded person and upon his request, a hearing will be held in the district court without a jury. Unless the retarded person or his representative objects, the hearing may be conducted without witnesses and the judge may enter judgment. If a hearing is requested and the retarded person does desire the appearance of witnesses, he is entitled to present evidence in his own behalf. The retarded person is likewise guaranteed the right to cross-examine witnesses who testify in support of the petition. Before the district court judge may enter an order requiring that the operation be performed, he must make the findings of fact required by § 35-43, which amounts to a judicial determination that the allegations contained in the petition are true.

[2] We construe this Section 43 to mean that the judge must find that the subject is likely to engage in sexual activity without using contraceptive devices and is therefore likely to impregnate or become impregnated. We derive that meaning from the clause of the statute saying ". . . because the person would be likely, unless sterilized, to procreate a child or children. . ." Although the phrase is not contained in the prior clause, it must have been the sense of the legislature to require only that which is necessary, and unless sexual activity or inability or unwillingness to utilize contraception is indicated by the evidence, there would be no occasion for resort to sterilization.

If the retarded person is dissatisfied with the outcome in the district court, an appeal as of right is available to the superior court for a trial de novo before a jury. The result in the superior court may be appealed through the normal appellate channels to the North Carolina Court of Appeals and to the North Carolina Supreme Court.

Section 35-45 establishes the retarded person's right to counsel and assures that this right must be protected "at all stages of the proceedings provided for herein." The statute provides for "*Miranda*-type" advice to the retarded person of entitlement to counsel at the time notice of the petition is given. Moreover, "this information shall be given in language and in a manner calculated to insure, insofar as such is possible in view of the individual's capability to comprehend it, that the recipient understands the entitlement." The retarded person is entitled to retain counsel, or, in the case of indigency, an attorney must be appointed.

The remaining sections of the statute govern the sterilization procedure after the court order has been entered, and presumably, affirmed, if appealed.

Other provisions of North Carolina law, which apply to civil proceedings generally, must also be regarded as applicable to proceedings under the sterilization statute. N.C. Gen. Stat. § 8-59 provides that the retarded person would have the ability to subpoena witnesses in his own behalf for proceedings before the district court. *See also* Rule 45, N.C. Rules of Civil Procedure, N.C. Gen. Stat. 1A-1. N.C. Gen. Stat. § 7A-198 provides for the reporting of all cases in the district court unless waived by consent of all parties, and N.C. Gen. Stat. § 7A-95 provides for similar reporting in the superior court. N.C. Gen. Stat. § 1-288 makes a transcript of the proceedings available to the retarded person, even if he is unable to pay the expense.

The statute does not contain any statement of the petitioner's burden of proof. But the North Carolina Supreme Court, in *In re Sterilization of Moore,* 289 N.C. 95, 221 S.E.2d 307 (1976), announced that "in keeping with the intent of the General Assembly, clearly expressed throughout the article, that the rights of the individual must be fully protected, we hold that evidence must be *clear, strong and convincing* before such an order may be entered." (Emphasis added.)

III

The United States as intervenor and the original plaintiff urge that we hold Article 7 of Chapter 35 of the North Carolina

General Statutes unconstitutional insofar as it provides for sterilization of mentally retarded persons. The reasons advanced are identical to those urged upon the North Carolina Supreme Court with respect to the same statute and rejected by that court in a carefully reasoned opinion by Mr. Justice Moore. *In re Moore, supra.*

[3-5] We hold that the legislative classification of mentally retarded persons is neither arbitrary nor capricious, but rests upon respectable medical knowledge and opinion that such persons are in fact different from the general population and may rationally be accorded different treatment for their benefit and the benefit of the public. Moreover, the classification is itself narrowed as to impact so that, as we interpret it, only mentally retarded persons who are sexually active, and unwilling or incapable of controlling procreation by other contraceptive means, *and* who are found to be likely to procreate a defective child, *or* who would be unable because of the degree of retardation to be able to care for a child, may be sterilized. The legislative dual purpose—to prevent the birth of a defective child or the birth of a nondefective child that cannot be cared for by its parent—reflects a compelling state interest and the classification rests upon a difference having a fair and substantial relation to the object of the legislation and does not, therefore, violate the Equal Protection Clause of the Fourteenth Amendment of the Constitution of the United States.

[6, 7] The traditional equal protection test is invidious discrimination. Indeed, the Supreme Court has often gone so far as to justify setting aside legislative classification "only if no grounds can be conceived to justify them." But the Court has also said that a statutory classification based upon suspect criteria or affecting fundamental rights will encounter equal protection difficulties unless justified by a compelling governmental interest. We think that all mentally retarded persons are sufficiently different from the general population to justify classification for some purposes without meeting the compelling governmental interest test. But we also think that

the right to procreate is a fundamental one and that under equal protection challenge sterilization cannot be ordered short of demonstrating a compelling governmental interest.

[8] We hold that the statute is not overly broad. Although it permits initiation of the sterilization procedure against any and all members of the class, it does *not* contemplate that all members of the class will be sterilized. Nor is the standard of selection so vague that it cannot be comprehended and applied. As we have made clear in our findings of fact, we are convinced that competent medical doctors and geneticists can predict in some cases with reasonable accuracy the likelihood of whether the parent will be able to care for his child. The burden of proof put upon the petitioner by the North Carolina Supreme Court that the evidence must be clear, strong and convincing strongly protects against predictive error and should effectively limit application of the statute to those members of the class within the stated legislative purpose. Failure to prove predictability would require, of course, denial of an order authorizing sterilization.

[9] For the reasons stated by Mr. Justice Moore for the Supreme Court of North Carolina, we hold that the statute is procedurally adequate to survive challenge under the Due Process Clause of the Fourteenth Amendment.

[10, 11] Finally we consider briefly the contention that the statute is invalid as a matter of "substantive" due process. We agree with the United States that the right to procreate is a fundamental right. As such it is protected by the Fourteenth Amendment's concept of personal autonomy and perhaps by other specific Amendments within the Bill of Rights. *See Roe* v. *Wade,* 410 U.S. 113, 93 S. Ct. 705; 35 L.Ed.2d. 147 (1973). The due process test of constitutionality of a statute that infringes upon a fundamental right is more than the ordinary one of a rational relationship to a valid state objective. To sustain this statute against substantive due process challenge it must be found that the state's interest is "compelling." We interpret Article 7 as narrowly drawn to express only the legitimate State interest of preventing the birth of a

defective child or the birth of a nondefective child that cannot be cared for by its parent, and that so viewed, the State's interest rises to the dignity of a compelling one. It would be otherwise had the State presumed to enact and implement that *all* mentally retarded persons should be sterilized. That is *not* the thrust of the statute.

By way of summary we hold that the entire statutory scheme embraced in Article 7 of Chapter 35, §§ 36-50, is constitutional except for subparagraph four of §39. We construe the statute to mean that a sterilization procedure may be initiated only by the director of the institution in which the retarded person resides or by the county director of social services. We further construe that statute to mean (§ 43) that before an order of sterilization can be entered, there must be a finding from evidence that is clear, strong and convincing that the subject is likely to engage in sexual activity without using contraceptive devices and that either a defective child is likely to be born or a child born that cannot be cared for by its parent. So construed, the statute is valid.

An appropriate judgment will be entered in accordance with this opinion.

STUMP ET AL. *V.* SPARKMAN ET VIR

CERTIORARI TO THE UNITED STATES COURT OF APPEALS FOR THE SEVENTH CIRCUIT

No. 76-1750. Argued January 10, 1978—
Decided March 28, 1978

OPINION OF THE COURT

Mr. JUSTICE WHITE delivered the opinion of the Court.

This case requires us to consider the scope of a judge's immunity from damages liability when sued under 42 U.S.C. §1983.

I

The relevant facts underlying respondents' suit are not in dispute. On July 9, 1971, Ora Spitler McFarlin, the mother of respondent Linda Kay Spitler Sparkman, presented to Judge Harold D. Stump of the Circuit Court of DeKalb County, Ind., a document captioned "Petition To Have Tubal Ligation Performed On Minor and Indemnity Agreement." The document had been drafted by her attorney, a petitioner here. In this petition Mrs. McFarlin stated under oath that her daughter was 15 years of age and was "somewhat retarded," although she attended public school and had been promoted each year with her class. The petition further stated that Linda had been associating with "older youth or young men" and had stayed out overnight with them on several occasions. As a result of this behavior and Linda's mental capabilities, it was stated that it would be in the daughter's best interest if she underwent a tubal ligation in order to "prevent unfortunate circumstances . . . ." In the same document Mrs. McFarlin also undertook to indemnify and hold harmless Dr. John Hines, who was to perform the operation, and the DeKalb Memorial Hospital, where the operation was to take place, against all causes of action that might arise as a result of the performance of the tubal ligation.

The petition was approved by Judge Stump on the same day. He affixed his signature as "Judge, DeKalb Circuit Court," to the statement that he did "hereby approve the above Petition by affidavit form on behalf of Ora Spitler McFarlin, to have Tubal Ligation performed upon her minor daughter, Linda Spitler, subject to said Ora Spitler McFarlin covenanting and agreeing to indemnify and keep indemnified Dr. John Hines and the DeKalb Memorial Hospital from any matters or causes of action arising therefrom."

On July 15, 1971, Linda Spitler entered the DeKalb Memorial Hospital, having been told that she was to have her appendix removed. The following day a tubal ligation was performed upon her. She was released several days later, unaware of the true nature of her surgery.

Approximately two years after the operation, Linda Spitler was married to respondent Leo Sparkman. Her inability to become pregnant led her to discover that she had been sterilized during the 1971 operation. As a result of this revelation, the Sparkmans filed suit in the United States District Court for the Northern District of Indiana against Mrs. McFarlin, her attorney, Judge Stump, and doctors who had performed and assisted in the tubal ligation, and the DeKalb Memorial Hospital. Respondents sought damages for the alleged violation of Linda Sparkman's constitutional rights; also asserted were pendent state claims for assault and battery, medical malpractice, and loss of potential fatherhood.

Ruling upon the defendants' various motions to dismiss the complaint, the District Court concluded that each of the constitutional claims asserted by respondents required a showing of state action and that the only state action alleged in the complaint was the approval by Judge Stump, acting as Circuit Court Judge, of the petition presented to him by Mrs. McFarlin. The Sparkmans sought to hold the private defendants liable on a theory that they had conspired with Judge Stump to bring about the allegedly unconstitutional acts. The District Court, however, held that no federal action would lie against any of the defendants because Judge Stump, the only state agent, was absolutely immune from suit under the doctrine of judicial immunity. The court stated that "whether or not Judge Stump's 'approval' of the petition may in retrospect appear to have been premised on an erroneous view of the law, Judge Stump surely had jurisdiction to consider the petition and to act thereon." *Sparkman* v. *McFarlin*, Civ. No. F 75-129 (ND Ind., May 13, 1976). Accordingly, under *Bradley* v. *Fisher*, 13 Wall. 335, 351 (1872), Judge Stump was entitled to judicial immunity.

On appeal, the Court of Appeals for the Seventh Circuit reversed the judgment of the District Court, holding that the "crucial issue" was "whether Judge Stump acted within his jurisdiction" and concluding that he had not. 552 F. 2d. at 174. He was accordingly not immune from damages liability under the controlling authorities. The Court of Appeals also held that the judge had forfeited his immunity "because of his failure to comply with elementary principles of procedural due process." *Id.*, at 176.

We granted certiorari, 434 U.S. 815 (1977), to consider the correctness of this ruling. We reverse.

II

The governing principle of law is well established and is not questioned by the parties. As early as 1872, the Court recognized that it was "a general principle of the highest importance to the proper administration of justice that a judicial officer, in exercising the authority vested in him, [should] be free to act upon his own convictions, without apprehension of personal consequences to himself." *Bradley* v. *Fisher, supra,* at 347. For that reason the Court held that "judges of courts of superior or general jurisdiction are not liable to civil actions for their judicial acts, even when such acts are in excess of their jurisdiction, and are alleged to have been done maliciously or corruptly.". . .

We cannot agree that there was a "clear absence of all jurisdiction" in the DeKalb County Circuit Court to consider the petition presented by Mrs. McFarlin. As an Indiana Circuit Court Judge, Judge Stump had "original exclusive jurisdiction in all cases at law and in equity whatsoever. . .," jurisdiction over the settlement of estates and over guardianships, appellate jurisdiction as conferred by law, and jurisdiction over "all other causes, matters and proceedings where exclusive jurisdiction thereof is not conferred by law upon some other court, board or officer." Ind. Code 33-4-4-3 (1975). This is indeed a broad jurisdictional grant; yet the Court of Appeals concluded that Judge Stump did not have jurisdiction over the petition authorizing Linda Sparkman's sterilization.

In doing so, the Court of Appeals noted that the Indiana statutes provided for the sterilization of institutionalized persons under certain circumstances, see Ind. Code §§ 16-13-13-1 through 16-13-13-4 (1973), but otherwise contained no express authority for judicial approval of tubal ligations. It is true that the statutory grant of general jurisdiction to the Indiana circuit courts does not itemize types of cases those courts may hear and hence does not expressly mention sterilization petitions presented by the parents of a minor. But in our view, it is more significant that there was no Indiana statute and no case law in 1971 prohibiting a circuit court, a court of general jurisdiction, from considering a petition of the type presented to Judge Stump. The statutory authority for the sterilization of institutionalized persons in the custody of the State does not warrant the inference that a court of general jurisdiction has no power to act on a petition for sterilization of a minor in the custody of her parents, particularly where the parents have authority under the Indiana statutes to "consent to and contract for medical or hospital care or treatment of [the minor] including surgery." Ind. Code § 16-8-4-2 (1973). The District Court concluded that Judge Stump had jurisdiction under § 33-4-4-3 to entertain and act upon Mrs. McFarlin's petition. We agree with the District Court, it appearing that neither by statute nor by case law has the board jurisdiction granted to the circuit courts of Indiana been circumscribed to foreclose consideration of a petition for authorization of a minor's sterilization.

The Court of Appeals also concluded that support for Judge Stump's actions could not be found in the common law of Indiana, relying in particular on the Indiana Court of Appeals' intervening decision in *A.L.* v. *G.R.H.*, 163 Ind. App. 636, 325 N.E. 2d. 501 (1975). In that case the Indiana court held that a parent does not have a common-law right to have a minor child sterilized, even though the parent might "sincerely believe the child's adulthood would benefit therefrom." The opinion, however, speaks only of the rights of the parents to consent to the sterilization of their child and does not question the *jurisdiction* of a circuit judge who is presented with such a petition from a parent. Although under that case a circuit judge would err as a matter of law if he were to approve a parent's petition seeking the sterilization of a child, the opinion in *A.L.* v. *G.R.H.* does not indicate that a circuit judge is without jurisdiction to entertain the petition. Indeed, the clear implication of the opinion is that, when presented with such a petition, the circuit judge should deny it on its merits rather than dismiss it for lack of jurisdiction. . . .

The fact that the issue before the judge is a controversial one is all the more reason that he should be able to act without fear of suit. As the Court pointed out in *Bradley:*

> Controversies involving not merely great pecuniary interests, but the liberty and character of the parties, and consequently exciting the deepest feelings, are being constantly determined

> in those courts, in which there is great conflict in the evidence and great doubt as to the law which should govern their decision. It is this class of cases which impose upon the judge the severest labor, and often create in his mind a painful sense of responsibility.

The Indiana law vested in Judge Stump the power to entertain and act upon the petition for sterilization. He is, therefore, under the controlling cases, immune from damages liability even if his approval of the petition was in error. Accordingly, the judgment of the Court of Appeals is reversed, and the case is remanded for further proceedings consistent with this opinion.

It is so ordered.

Index

MIX
Papier aus verantwortungsvollen Quellen
Paper from responsible sources
FSC® C105338

If you have any concerns about our products,
you can contact us on
ProductSafety@springernature.com

In case Publisher is established outside the EU,
the EU authorized representative is:
Springer Nature Customer Service Center GmbH
Europaplatz 3, 69115 Heidelberg, Germany

Printed by Libri Plureos GmbH
in Hamburg, Germany